"As a physician well versed in nutrition, I have maintained a healthful lifestyle, so I was somewhat skeptical at the onset about this nutritional journey. I attended Karyn's class weekly, and I implemented her doctrine daily as instructed. Her teaching style and methods were relaxed yet pointed. Her explanation of the science of raw eating was sensible and logical. Her conclusions, based on years of formal study and observations in the human laboratory, were reliable. From a nutritional standpoint, all of the elements of a healthful diet can be attained through raw vegan eating because nature in its simplest state provides everything we need to survive.

Throughout the course, many students experienced and openly shared significant health improvements. Illnesses such as arthritis, diabetes, high blood pressure, and joint pain became less symptomatic. I saw my blood pressure decrease significantly, and I lost several pounds. I no longer had doubts about the program. Almost everyone experienced weight loss and felt empowered after gaining control of their health journey and longevity. I highly endorse Karyn's classes and her ideals. Through her research and personal experience, she has become one of the foremost experts in this expanding science. I am honored to be her student and friend."

William D. Yates, MD, FACS

"One of the most important things I have learned in my twenty years of trying to help patients improve their health is that to be well, one must nourish well, breathe well, move well, relate well, and detoxify well. I have known Karyn for many years, and I consider her to be one of the best living examples of this

philosophy. She has been an inspiration for me and thousands of people who want to feel better. Her vibrance serves as testimony to the benefits of eating living food and avoiding and removing toxins."

Carlos M. Reynes, MD

"I was initially introduced to 'Karyn's raw law' twelve plus years ago after having been a practicing dentist for ten years. I was blasted with new information that challenged my myopia, and I found it expedient to reassess some things that I had learned in dental school. Over the years, my personal health and health IQ have continually escalated as the result of meeting this superb teacher, Karyn Calabrese. I have enjoyed personal consultations and detoxification classes, and I continue to detox to this day. During detoxification, I never tire of good news, small miracles, and testimonies. I'm elated by testimonies of people who no longer have to take medications.

I have experienced an awakening, and I can't go back. I know too much. As we awaken, we become the people we are supposed to be. Sincerest thanks and gratitude for my ever-growing awakening."

Yvette Collins, DDS

SOAK YOUR NUTS

CLEANSING WITH KARYN

Karyn Calabrese

BOOK PUBLISHING COMPANY
Summertown Tennessee

Library of Congress Cataloging-in-Publication Data

Calabrese, Karyn.
    Soak your nuts : cleansing with Karyn / Karyn Calabrese.
        p. cm.
    Includes index.
    ISBN 978-1-57067-264-4
    1. Raw food diet.   2. Detoxification (Health)   I. Title.
    RM237.5.C27 2011
    613.2'65—dc22

                                           2010051254

Cover and interior design: John Wincek
Cover photography: Mike Roberts
Food photography: Lin Eagle

Book Publishing Company
P.O. Box 99
Summertown, TN 38483
888-260-8458
www.bookpubco.com

ISBN: 978-1-57067-264-4

Book Publishing Company is a member of Green Press Initiative. We chose to print this title on paper with 100% post consumer recycled content, processed without chlorine, which saved the following natural resources:

    40 trees
    1,101 pounds of solid waste
    18.126 gallons of water
    3,764 pounds of greenhouse gases
    13 million BTU of energy

For more information on Green Press Initiative, visit www.greenpressinitiative.org.

Environmental impact estimates were made using the Environmental Defense Fund Paper Calculator. For more information, visit www.papercalculator.org.

Printed on recycled paper

17 16 15 14 13 12 11   9 8 7 6 5 4 3 2

contents

To my son, Secondino "Dino" Giuseppe Calabrese

1970–2008

In one of the stars I shall be living. In one of them I shall be laughing,
and so it will be as if all the stars were laughing when you look at the sky at night.

ANTOINE DE SAINT-EXUPÉRY, *THE LITTLE PRINCE*

acknowledgments

I must start by thanking my mother for giving me the secret to life long before *The Secret* was a household phenomenon, before people learned to believe that their spoken word became their reality. She taught me early on that a mistake had been made with the utterance and usage of the word "can't." No such word exists. Consequently, it never occurred to me that I can't do, accomplish, or create anything meaningful I choose, including establishing the longest-standing raw-food restaurant in the country. Even before raw foods were so well-known or received, it never occurred to me to measure my success in dollars—the success was in what I created. My mother also taught me that creating beauty from within was everlasting and to always put myself in someone else's shoes before judging. All these valuable lessons have helped to move me along my journey of self-love, spirituality, health, and service to others.

Thank you to my children, Dino, Nicole, and Michael, and my grandchildren, Quinton and Emilio, for giving me the chance to experience unconditional love from and through them. For helping to teach and remind me that God's children are on their own course to create the meaning of their lives—an invaluable tool for me in teaching the thousands that have gone through this journey with me. In addition, I give my love and thanks to Mitch (my dog) and Maliku (my cat).

And last but far from least, thank you to my life partner, husband, best friend, protector, supporter, and living Buddha, who has steadfastly supported all my dreams physically, emotionally, financially, and unconditionally. This support has allowed my vision of helping others find their own healing journey to come to life. Jerry Scherer—all of us on this journey owe you.

And thank you one and all for coming into my life either through my classes, restaurants, lectures, products, or this book. Whatever I've done that has sparked your interest of self-renewal, no matter how large or small, thank you for the time you've trusted in me and invested in yourself. I thank you from the bottom of my heart for making this a better world for all of us by sharing in a vision to awaken and heal. For as we all know, if you don't take care of your body—the most magnificent machine you'll ever be given—where will you live?

foreword

It is with great honor and respect that I write words of praise for Karyn Calabrese's *Soak Your Nuts*. Her newest offering to the realm of loving raw foodism will indeed inspire you to understand what it means to accept the gift of vitality and know thyself.

For many years, Karyn has represented and practiced the timeless truths that create ageless beauty, health, intelligence, abundance, and consciousness. Over a quarter century ago, I met Karyn at the Reverend Ann Wigmore's center in Boston, Massachusetts. Others besides Rev. Ann at that time attempted raw-food detoxification and became self-proclaimed "experts," endorsing a wide array of directives that did not work in the long run. Many tried to copy her—but no one had the magic of Rev. Ann, who always spoke of Karyn as her protégé. How prophetic she was. Now it is very easy to see where the student excels the teacher with all her glowing acts and deeds!

Ever since the time of our first meeting, Karyn and I have joined energies to make the world a better place for all future generations. I have tremendous gratitude for my relationship with Karyn as well as all the workshops she has organized for me.

Karyn is like a fine wine, matured with age and yet eternally youthfull. She truly opens her heart to share her experiences and passion for health. She has constantly demonstrated her knowledge of *The Secret* within her wide influence in Chicago, and now she is blazing her trail through the infinite digital world. She walks her talk, which is certainly

more like a sacred, cosmic dance. So many have been touched and deeply cleansed by her guidance and example.

I have been lecturing all over the United States and have eaten in most of the raw-food restaurants. Karyn's raw fine-dining meals, as well as the deli, stand out among all the rest. With *Soak Your Nuts*, you will have Karyn sitting you down to share what all of Chicago has been "rawing" about. It is the book that will keep you vegan and excite you to make deliciously delightful raw food while healing yourself wherever you may need it—whether you have too much fat, a joy deficiency, low energy, or even cancer.

The cleansing and detoxing programs explained in this book are amazing. Karyn's life's work has always emphasized the importance of optimal health with long-term results, and you are now the fortunate recipient of her wisdom. Embrace the principles in *Soak your Nuts* and, just like Karyn, you'll discover the wonders of peace, health, and beauty within and without.

With love in service,

REV. VIKTORAS KULVINSKAS, MS

co-founder of the Hippocrates Health Institute
and author of *Survival in the 21st Century*

rules for being human

1. You will receive a body. You may like it or hate it, but it will be yours for the duration of this lifetime.

2. You are enrolled in a full-time informal school called life. You will learn lessons. Each day in this school you have the opportunity to learn them. You may like the lessons or think them irrelevant and stupid.

3. There are no mistakes. Only lessons. Growth is a process of trial and error experimentation. The 'failed' experiments are as much a part of the process as the experiment that ultimately 'works.'

4. A lesson is repeated until it is learned. A lesson will be presented to you in various forms until you have learned it. When you have learned it, you can then go on to the next one.

5. Learning lessons does not end. There is no part of life that does not contain lessons. If you are alive, there are lessons to be learned.

6. "There" is no better than "here." When "there" has become a "here," you will simply obtain another "there" that will again look better than "here."

7. Others are merely mirrors of you. You cannot love or hate something about another person unless it reflects to you something you love or hate about yourself.

8. What you make of your life is up to you. You have all the tools and resources you need. What you do with them is up to you. The choice is yours.

9. Your answers lie inside of you. The answers to life's questions lie inside of you. All you need to do is look, listen and trust.

10. You will forget all this . . . over and over again!

—AUTHOR UNKNOWN

introduction
A BEAUTIFUL LIFE

We've all heard the saying "If it seems too good to be true, it probably is." Nowhere is this warning more relevant than in the sphere of health and wellness. Although Americans spend more money per capita in pursuit of good health than people in any other developed country, we remain obese and increasingly prone to chronic and degenerative illness. We look for solutions on grocery store shelves, which groan under the weight of deceptively unhealthful fat-free and vitamin-enriched products. We seek quick fixes by popping a rainbow of pills to control our cholesterol and stress levels and cure our every ill. And still we continue to feel just plain lousy.

Even those of us who consider ourselves to be disease free suffer from allergies, colon and bowel disturbances, fluctuations in blood sugar, headaches, indigestion, low metabolism, obesity, sinus problems, skin conditions, and a host of aches and pains. Over time, we have become accustomed to feeling under the weather. We have come to accept problematic symptoms and that tired, dragged-out feeling of general malaise. That blah feeling, we tell ourselves, is our lot in life.

Because we are a certain age or gender or ethnicity, because we swam in from a particular gene pool, or because we, as a culture, are prone to a host of maladies brought about by the physical and emotional stresses of modern life, we simply can't expect to feel well—or can we? The truth is that we can. At well past sixty, I am living proof. And so are the countless others whose longevity and quality of life have been utterly transformed by the revitalizing power of living food and detoxification.

This was my first class with Karyn and I will never be the same! I lost 8 pounds. I feel lighter, happier and have a clearer vision about life in general. I see a long, wonderful road ahead Thank you, Karyn. —E. N.

MIRACLES AND OTHER EVERYDAY OCCURRENCES

Consider Maria. Maria came to my health center in the spring of 1998. A forty-five-year-old executive secretary working in Chicago, Maria had suffered from extreme digestive problems for fifteen years. During that time, she had visited numerous physicians who provided her with a range of diagnoses, including spastic colon, irritable bowel syndrome, chronic fatigue syndrome, and nervous stomach. Although Maria tried the treatments suggested by the doctors, the slightest tension or stress always put her stomach in a painful twist. She couldn't get through a day without steadily consuming antacids.

During our first meeting, it became clear to me that Maria had come to view her problem in much the same way as her doctors did: as a localized condition. If Maria's stomach hurt, then her problem was clearly confined to her digestive tract. Right? Wrong! I explained to Maria that human beings are not machines made up of cogs and widgets. Our "parts" function not only in synergy with each other but also in response to our emotions, thoughts, and feelings. So, our first step was to identify any emotional issues that might be causing or exacerbating her symptoms. Second, we replaced Maria's standard American diet with an eating program that would restore her health. I asked Maria to eliminate dairy products, meat, chicken, and fish from her diet and begin to incorporate the raw and living foods that restore health from the cellular level up.

My skin is clearer. I have great mental clarity. My clothing fits better. In general, I feel better than I have felt in the past six years. This program has given me the tools and the knowledge that I need to finally take control of my health and become the captain of my fate. I'm so happy that I participated in this program! It was a great experience!
—D. H.

In a matter of weeks, Maria looked and felt like a new person. Filled with energy and glowing with vibrant health, she was totally symptom free for the first time in more than a decade. She could eat, work, and live without fear of sudden gastric symptoms. Maria had completely eliminated any sign of her "illness," something the top doctors in Chicago had been unable to do.

Best of all, she had taken on a new sense of confidence. Her skin was supple and her eyes were bright and clear. Her youthful beauty and energy propelled her into an exciting new phase of life. Physically and psychically, she was restored. Maria's friends couldn't help but consider Maria's transformation a miracle. Like most Americans, they weren't accustomed to seeing such dramatic changes as the result of nonsurgical rejuvenation techniques.

Yet, what happened to Maria was no miracle. It was simply the fulfillment of nature's promise to us all: if we live in alignment with Mother Nature's plan, if we stop filling our bodies with toxins and start eating the healing, revitalizing

foods we were intended to eat, we can look well, feel well, and *be* well as long as we live. Inner healing and outer beauty are within our reach. The real miracle may be that any of us survives years of eating processed foods laden with additives and preservatives, breathing polluted air, drinking chemically treated water, and enduring the side effects of unnecessary medications and the hundreds of poisons we encounter every day.

I am as lithe and lean as a greyhound.

My armpits smell like celery.

— Anonymous

As Maria discovered, foods are powerful healers that can restore us, body and soul. Maria's story is not unique. In over three decades of work as a wellness counselor, I have seen thousands of men and women relieve a host of conditions, including depressed metabolism, digestive problems, fatty tumors, fibromyalgia, headaches, insulin dependence, obesity, sinus problems, uterine fibroids, and many chronic and degenerative illnesses. They are able to do so because they are willing to partake in the cycles of renewal that energize and constantly transform every natural creature and element on this wonderful planet.

YOUR BEAUTIFUL LIFE BEGINS HERE

In the chapters that follow, I outline an effective 28-day program that I call Nature's Healing System, a transformational journey to boundless energy, radiant health, and lifelong vitality. This program is really about cause and effect. Every action, every decision, every manmade intervention with nature, has a consequence. I believe there is a certain way we were meant to live and to eat for optimum health. When we do so, we are more likely to be free from disease and fulfilled in body, mind, and spirit.

I am introducing you to a natural healing process that will remove years of accumulated toxins from your body more effectively than any other program or product I know of. No matter what your physical condition, no matter how much willpower you believe you do or do not have, you can cleanse your body, look years younger, and prolong your life by following the natural, nourishing detoxification program described in this book.

Do these promises seem hard to believe? I encourage you to decide for yourself after reading the honest

Why Soak Your Nuts?

After your initial chuckle, I'm sure many of you are wondering why in the world I called my book *Soak Your Nuts*. I have a good explanation. Soaked nuts have a practical application in raw-food preparation. When nuts are soaked in water for a few hours, an enzyme inhibitor is broken down, allowing the nutrients in the nuts to be more easily digested and absorbed. When you increase nutrient absorption, you will be satisfied more quickly and less likely to plow through a whole bag of nuts in one sitting.

I also used this title because I want to remind you to keep a sense of humor during the detoxification process. I'm asking you to do things you may never have heard of or thought you would be capable of doing, and laughter definitely helps ease the fear and tension. If we take ourselves too seriously, the cleansing process can become burdensome when it should be a joyful journey. The symptoms of cleansing can sometimes be uncomfortable, but keeping a positive attitude and sense of humor can help you manage them and come out better than ever on the other side.

and often astounding testimonials in this book. They are from people who have invested just four weeks in an easy-to-follow nutritional program and reaped a lifetime of benefits. They are the words of people who set their own evolution in motion and are now utterly changed, inside and out.

Beyond the many internal changes you will experience while participating in the program, you will see a new you on the outside. You will see the clear, youthful skin of a reawakened body, energized from deep within. In your clear eyes, you will see the glowing reflection of a regenerating self—a body in balance, a soul on the brink of its own discovery. Your more fulfilling and beautiful life begins today. Welcome it!

Our deepest fear is not that we are inadequate.

Our deepest fear is that we are powerful beyond measure.

It is our light, not our darkness, that most frightens us.

We ask ourselves, who am I to be brilliant, gorgeous, talented, fabulous?

Actually who are you not to be?

You are a child of God. Your playing small does not serve the world.

There is nothing enlightening about shrinking so that other people won't feel unsure around you.

We were born to make manifest the glory of God that is within us.

It is not just in some of us; it is in everyone.

As we let our own light shine, we unconsciously give other people permission to do the same.

As we are liberated from our own fear, our presence automatically liberates others.

Marianne Williamson

Presented by Nelson Mandela in his 1994 inaugural speech

Karyn's detox program works! If you follow her instructions and stay focused on your goals, you will experience success. —R. W.

If you had told me ten years ago that I'd be eating only raw food, I would have said, "What the hell are you smoking?" But if you want to rocket your life to a positive, powerful place, do the detox and cleanse. Your body and mind will be better for it. —J. M.

This is my third raw-food detox class in the last twelve months. Each fast has been beneficial in different ways and has opened me up to greater healing possibilities. I have gained confidence in the control I have over my own health and healing. —M. K.

About two years ago my doctor told me that I was diabetic. My blood sugar has never been under 120; in fact, I would really get excited when it was below 130. Since I started the detox class, however, my blood sugar has been under 100. In fact, today it was 91. Thank you, thank you! I've shared my journey with many family members, friends, and associates, and they are all very proud of my success and want to experience the detox for themselves. Most of all, I'm proud of my accomplishments and that I have changed my life in a very positive way. —P. H.

I didn't think I could ever do this—four weeks of meatless, breadless, butterless existence—but I did. Now here I am, several pounds lighter, with thicker hair, stronger nails, and no more sinus or skin problems. —I. A. C.

My intention for taking the class was to cleanse my body and mind and learn as much as I could about nutrition. What was most amazing for me was to experiment with when and how much I ate. I realized what a small amount was required to satisfy my appetite and cravings, and I no longer feel a need to eat from the time I get up to the time I go to bed. The detox affirmed how strong the mind and body can be. And I had fun doing it! If you told me thirty days ago how good I would feel now or that I would accomplish what I did, I would not have believed you. —M. M.

I am an average thirty-five-year-old male, who had extremely high cholesterol and a family history of heart disease. I had no excuse not to take Karyn's class and do whatever was required. I ended up losing my chronic headaches and excess weight, lowering my cholesterol dramatically, and getting off medication. To my surprise, my energy level increased significantly and my sleep improved. But what I never expected was the peace of mind I gained! —J. K.

I came to the detox class because, at 44, I felt old. My skin and hair were dull, and my body ached and felt heavy. I had lost my femininity. Now I feel that I am coming back. I am lighter and focused. I am amazed at the power my body holds. I am prepared to care for the inside of me as well as the outside. When I was brushing my hair this morning, it dawned on me that I have found love—love for myself— and it has surrounded me. —L. W.

cleanse
NATURE'S HEALING SYSTEM

The May 5, 2000, episode of the *Oprah Winfrey Show* featured a topic that piqued the interest, roused the hopes, and stirred the curiosity of millions of people. The focus of that show was how ordinary men and women could discover the secrets of agelessness, that elusive mixture of physical vitality, lively intelligence, and overall youthfulness that define timeless beauty. There can be no surprise that the show was memorable for so many viewers. After all, human beings have been searching for the

secret of eternal youth for thousands of years. And here, in Chicago, Oprah rounded up a group of remarkably well-preserved people whose very existence seemed to defy the idea that aging means getting sick and wrinkled.

At age fifty-three, I was one of Oprah's guests, one of the lucky few who seemed to have beaten the clock. Ironically, thirty years before that show, no one would have predicted that I would become the poster child for anything but lousy genes and deteriorating health. In fact, any doctor who knew my family history might be shocked to see me alive and well, let alone the picture of health and an inspiration to others.

I was born in 1947 to a father who didn't stick around to change diapers and a young mother who was a free spirit, unencumbered by life's demands and, in some ways, less than responsible. By the age of ten, I had grown into a sickly child, prone to allergies and sensitive to a host of foods and products. As a teenager, it was not unusual for me to smoke a cigarette, follow it with a big greasy hamburger, and then wash it all down with four or five sodas. It's an understatement to say that vegetarianism was not a part of my young life. I was always tired and often moody and, unlike my happy-go-lucky parent, I saw little joy in life.

Since my mother's life was unstructured and nomadic, so was mine. Although she loved me, my adventurous, open-minded mother took poor care of herself and kept a very loose rein on me. By the time I became a young adult, the

effects of my slipshod diet had begun to take a toll. I suffered from acne, cystic breasts, and chronic constipation and other digestive problems. Looking back, I am sure now that this lifestyle would have led me to an early grave if destiny—my mother's and my own—hadn't intervened.

When I was twenty-seven, my forty-seven-year-old mother was diagnosed with facial cancer. Being the lifelong seeker that she was, she began to search for alternative routes to healing. She discovered the power of nature's medicines, including botanical remedies, herbal treatments, and juicing.

Seven months after her diagnosis, my mother died from complications brought about by chemotherapy. Nevertheless, her search for wellness delivered me from my ailments. Even though the vitamin- and nutrient-laden juices she made could not protect her from the negative effects of chemotherapy, they settled my stomach and cleared my skin. The herbs she took could not compensate for the prescription drugs that weakened her body, but they made me strong. For the first time, the systems of my body began working in unison. I felt better, I looked better, and I wanted to learn more about the healing power of vegetables—and about my place in the world of natural healing.

Shortly after I began my transformational health journey, a doctor diagnosed me with appendicitis and ordered me into the hospital. I refused to have the operation. Instead, I checked myself out and immersed myself in books on natural remedies. After several days of holistic therapy, the pains went away, never to return.

During this cleanse, I have accomplished more than I thought I would. I have lost 6½ pounds and feel more energetic, and my blood pressure has gone down. Karyn said that the body was designed to last 120 years or more. Dare I hope for another fifty-nine? —E. C.

My healing voyage was well under way. My body had already shown me that it felt better and worked better when I stopped eating animal-based foods like dairy products, meat, chicken, and fish. My health really began to blossom when I chose to eat raw, living food. That's when my journey took its most significant turn. I discovered Ann Wigmore, the pioneer nutritionist and advocate of living food who founded the Hippocrates Health Institute. Her students affectionately called her Dr. Wigmore. Under her mentoring, I learned the importance of raw food and detoxification. As they say, when the student is ready, the teacher appears. I had found both my guru and a belief system.

Thinking about it now, I see that I could have very easily followed my mother's path. I experimented with alcohol, drugs, smoking, and the same free-spirited lifestyle. My dysfunctional childhood certainly lent itself to a dysfunctional adulthood. Fortunately, I was blessed with a strong will to survive, deep spirituality, and knowledgeable guides, who appeared just when I needed them most.

Although I have faced many crises in my life—including a bad marriage, homelessness, and a lack of resources to feed my children—I have always remained positive. I also began to nourish and nurture my body. I know that if I take care of the miraculous body and mind that God gave me, I will always have shelter from life's challenges. I will never be truly homeless.

When people meet me they assume I must descend from a robust gene pool. That's what the people in Oprah's audience thought. Nothing could be further from the truth. My mother died at age forty-eight, my grandmother at fifty, and my great-grandmother at sixty. Although their early deaths could be interpreted as ominous signs for me, I believe I will live well past one hundred without suffering from debilitating illness, but obviously not because I have any genetic advantage. Rather, I expect to attain longevity through my consistent practice of detoxifying, inside and out, at least four times a year. I have built a strong body that will allow me to remain healthy as I age.

Now in my sixties, I have the stamina of a woman half my age. My diet has evolved from vegetarian to vegan to raw vegan. I eat mainly green vegetables, fruits, sea vegetables, sprouted seeds, sprouted grains, and, of course, the soaked nuts I refer to in this book's title. I use supplements and drink fresh vegetable juices. In an average day, 70 percent of the food I consume is chlorophyll rich. This is important, because chlorophyll delivers oxygen to the cells, strengthens muscle tissue, and removes waste. I cannot overstate the value of a chlorophyll-rich diet.

A few of the things I have achieved over the last few weeks include clarity, balance, the satisfaction of knowing I can accomplish whatever goals I set for myself, and a true sense of self-reliance. In addition, I'm much more aware and concerned about what I'm putting into my body. This program is a great catalyst for anyone interested in improving his or her health and life. —J. T.

The benefits of my diet and lifestyle allow me to enjoy life fully. I wear the same dress size I wore as a teenager. I practice yoga and ballet regularly. I have never suffered from cramps, depression, or headaches, and I went through menopause without any of the typical symptoms, including hot flashes. And I have achieved all this despite my and my family's dismal medical histories.

I have been a health advocate for over thirty-five years. During that time, I have coached thousands of people back to vitality by teaching them the fundamentals of good health. Most people believe there is some big secret to staying healthy. But if there is any secret to looking and feeling your best, it is simply this: your body and nature must work together as a team. When they do not, when your physical self is out of alignment with what nature intended, the result is illness and disease.

The most effective way to realign your body with the wisdom of nature is by clearing away the built-up toxins that prevent you from getting the most benefit

from your food, make you susceptible to illness, and smother your stamina. That means cleansing and detoxifying, gently and efficiently.

AGELESS WISDOM, NEW HOPE

Today, nearly every culture and religious group maintains a cleansing or fasting ritual to rid the body of impurities and focus the mind beyond the physical here and now. Many cultures do it the way their ancient ancestors did. Native Americans do it in sweat tepees. The Japanese do it in communal steam baths. Those who follow ayurveda, the five-thousand-year-old Indian system of healing, do it by fasting and taking herbs to increase the digestive fire and burn away *ama*, the toxic residue that results from an improper diet. So as you are reading this, no doubt up to your chemically deodorized armpits in impurities and wondering whether you might benefit from a cleanse, I encourage you not to overlook five thousand years of historical evidence.

Although some of us may look upon cleansing rituals as quaint throwbacks to a more spiritual or even a more superstitious time, the truth is that we are in greater need of cleansing now than ever before. Even when the world was far less polluted, cleansing was traditionally regarded as a normal, healthful, and necessary part of life. It is an important way to respond to what your body is telling you. Discomfort and disease are the body's way of screaming at us to wake up, get rid of what it can't use, and start giving it what it needs.

We are subject to toxins from many sources. The one we have the most control over is our food. Many of us hold the misconception that we are eating more healthful foods than we did in the past. After all, modern processed foods are fat free, low fat, and sugar free (yet miraculously taste sweet), right? Look closer. You need only check ingredient lists to see that these artificially colored, flavored, and preserved foods are hardly modern-day manna. Fat-free foods are laden with chemicals that give them mouth appeal, and most packaged foods are full of fillers and void of nutrients. Your body is not benefiting from these foods. In fact, you might as well be eating the cardboard packaging!

Over thirty years ago I adopted a raw vegan diet, which many would consider to be close to perfect. In addition, I don't smoke, drink, or take drugs. And yet, even though 99.9 percent of the food I eat is raw and I avoid unhealthful habits, I

What Is a Raw Vegan Diet?

My unique cleansing program, Nature's Healing System, is based on a raw vegan diet. "Raw" means uncooked foods, or foods that are not cooked above 118 degrees Fahrenheit (48 degrees Celsius). "Vegan" means no food of animal origin, such as dairy products, eggs, meat, chicken, or fish. What's left, you may ask? A bountiful array of delicious, enzyme-rich foods and drinks, including vegetables, fruits, sprouts, nuts, seeds, sea vegetables, and fresh juices. See a small sampling of recipes in chapter 6 (pages 105 to 116) and a list of raw-food recipe books in Resources (page 119).

still detox a minimum of four times a year. Why? Because I live in the real world and not on a mountaintop or in a rainforest. I get my clothes dry cleaned, drive behind buses, and run businesses. In other words, I am bombarded by chemicals, environmental pollutants, and all kinds of stressors in my physical environment and daily life. Having seen the way these factors take a toll on my well-being despite my optimal diet, I can't imagine how people function when they consume coffee, dairy products, fast food, red meat, and soda on a daily basis. Trust me, if I need detoxification, everyone does!

WHY CLEANSE?

Alternative practitioners and open-minded physicians recommend detoxification to treat a host of chronic conditions and symptoms, including allergies, asthma, cancer, congestion, degenerative diseases, fatigue, fever, joint pain, skin problems, and more. If you have a chronic illness, you may well find the symptoms of that illness diminished after your cleanse. I believe that arthritis, arteriosclerosis, cancer, chronic fatigue syndrome, multiple sclerosis, type 2 diabetes, and other degenerative diseases can be prevented, lessened in intensity, or eradicated entirely if we provide our natural healing systems with the proper fuel. Over the years, I have worked with people who suffered from a variety of health conditions, including cancer and AIDS. Detoxification has been the solution to their health problems. I have seen many of them reduce their suffering and go into remission.

The activist and comedian Dick Gregory has said, "Man does not die; he kills himself with his fork." I encourage participants in my 28-day program to make new food choices and introduce more nurturing foods to their bodies. During and after the cleanse, you will find that your body will crave a different type of food than it did before you detoxified. That's because detoxification clears away years of built-up poisons and allows your body to show you its natural preference for nourishing food. Follow your body's inclinations. The healthy cravings of a pure body will lead you to a better way of eating and living. The good food you eat will nourish your soul and restore nature's gift of healing. You will trim off excess weight, become invigorated, and slow the aging process. So you see, not all cravings are bad!

The good news is this: the human body was designed to heal itself. Whatever your age, whatever your condition, if you give your body what it needs to look and

Your Creator of Choice

I frequently refer to God in this book, and I want to take the chance here to make one important clarification. As an earnest student and lover of all world religions and spiritual traditions, I know that the definition of God is different for each of us. For me, God is the force that creates and sustains us. Some of you may revere many gods or none at all. Or you may equate God with nature, spirit, or even the wonderful complexity of biology. Whatever your beliefs, the point I want to make is that this book is not about a specific religion or spiritual tradition. When I mention God, I ask you to use your own interpretation, applying the term in any way that resonates with you.

The Three Rs

To let my students know what to expect from my cleansing program, I introduce it by using what I call the Three Rs:

Remove the foods and chemicals that are depressing your metabolism, undermining your body's ability to function, and compromising your health.

Replace those harmful foods and chemicals with the healthful foods that completely nourish your biological systems, from the cellular level up.

Rebalance your eating, your thinking, and your habits to build the youthful, vital body you were meant to enjoy.

feel its best, you will not only extend your life but also dramatically improve the quality of your life. Nature's Healing System provides you with the tools you need to rebuild your physical vigor by cleaning away toxins that can undermine your health. Within days, any feeling of lethargy (the kind of general malaise I've come to call "twenty-first century syndrome") will become nothing more than a dull memory. And because your body will no longer have to exhaust its life force digesting food that it was never meant to encounter, it can begin the wondrous work of healing. Like many other people who have gone through my cleansing program, you may find that conditions you never thought would go away begin to turn around. You'll feel better, look better, and function the way you did years ago. Before you know it, your clothes will begin to fit differently, and your skin will take on a youthful glow that you thought was as long gone as the corsage from your senior prom.

WHAT IS CLEANSING?

What does detoxification mean in terms of this cleanse? Most of us associate the term "detox" with rehabilitation programs for users of drugs or alcohol. For our purpose, detoxing means bringing balance to our bodies by cleansing them of the cumulative effects of any number of inefficient fuels and environmental toxins, and restoring them to optimal health. I call my program Nature's Healing System because we are truly healing by living as God and nature intended.

Many of us don't think about cleansing our insides, even though we take care of external injuries right away. We all know that when you cut your finger and clean the wound, your skin will repair itself. In a couple of days, you won't be able to tell that you ever had a scratch. No harm done. But if you expose the wound to dirt and bacteria, it will fester and become infected. If left untreated, the infection might escalate into a problem that is too large for your body's defenses to fight. It could even develop into a chronic condition or disease.

I want you to think of detoxifying in a similar way. Although we think of our bodies as unassailable fortresses that defend us, the fact is that our skin, our lungs, and our digestive tracts are continuously assaulted by all manner of dangerous toxins that we take in, often without thinking about it. If we don't clean

our bodies from the inside out, these toxins will increase and injure us. Over time, our injuries will worsen—just like an untreated wound.

The 28-day program outlined in this book is a powerful but gentle cleansing system I have developed over many years. It pulls toxins from the digestive tract, your body's tissues, and even your cells by

- combating excess acid and bringing your body to a more balanced state,
- eliminating overgrowths of yeast, also called candida, in your body (numerous health conditions can develop in people who have yeast overgrowths),
- penetrating and loosening the years-old layers of mucus that line your colon and make it difficult for you to absorb and use nutrients efficiently, and
- providing your body with revitalizing oxygen, which is the building block of the strong, healthy cells that are necessary for detoxification.

In my opinion, an unbalance in any of these areas leads to most, if not all, allergies, deficiencies, and diseases, including cancer. Vibrant health can be restored only when all the body's systems work together at optimum strength.

TOXINS

We need to detox now more than ever. Our bodies are constantly trying to reach a state of balance as they are under attack by inefficient foods and environmental toxins. We breathe off some of these toxins if our lungs are not damaged from years of smoking or exposure to pollution. We eliminate other toxins in our urine, feces, and sweat if our digestive processes are working efficiently and we aren't clogging our sweat glands with antiperspirants. However, in our chemically toxic world, where it is the norm to eat processed foods, use prescription drugs, and live and work in sick buildings in polluted cities, we may take in more toxins than our bodies can handle.

Toxic Foods

Detoxification doesn't just mean removing the toxins that have already taken up residence in your body; it also means making a conscious effort to stop putting in new impurities. To cleanse effectively enough to reach the layers of poisons built up inside the intestines, we must stop trying to live on the foods that keep us from fully living. We take in bushel baskets of impurities through our food, including the foods we choose specifically because we believe they are supposed to be healthful. Yet some of these foods are highly processed and taste terrible. Have you ever eaten a rice cake? What are they really made of? Styrofoam packing peanuts?

When we choose what "fuel" goes into our bodies, we are influenced by a multitude of factors other than hunger, such as the time of day, the kind of food that is readily available, our state of mind, our energy level, and our social obligations. As a result, we often eat for the wrong reasons and put substances into our bodies that do more harm than good. Most of the food in our grocery stores and on our pantry shelves is not the appropriate fuel for our bodies. Even those of us who would never put the wrong fuel in our cars add chemical sludge to our bodies every day. Is it so unthinkable that, after years of this behavior, we might need to clean out the tank?

Your body was built to operate optimally on the fuel nature provides: nutritious foods that draw their power from the earth. These are the foods that nourish our cells; these are the foods that heal. Needless to say, if we feast on these foods the way nature intended—at the peak of freshness, brimming with vitamins and minerals—we allow our bodies to channel the earth's God-given power to restore itself. After years of eating foods that put your body in an unbalanced state, you may not initially enjoy some of the natural healing foods I'm recommending; in fact, you may detest them. Unfortunately, the less you like something, the more you may need it. The process of bringing the body back into balance isn't always smooth and symptom free.

At first, your diet change may bring about some interesting symptoms. As impurities are released into your bloodstream, urine, and feces, you may experience some "cleansing reactions" to these toxins. These reactions can range from headaches to flulike symptoms, or even strange metallic or medicinal tastes in your mouth. Regardless of the number and severity of your cleansing reactions, you will certainly become aware of an increase in energy. And you will feel noticeably less hungry. While these reactions may be temporarily uncomfortable, pushing through this phase will bring you great rewards. Think of your cleansing reactions as blessings.

Cleansing reactions are typically followed by an up-and-at-'em feeling, which means that you have cleared your digestive tract enough to enhance your body's ability to absorb nutrients from your food. This feeling of renewal, revitaliza-

Enzymes: The Life Force

As the naturopath and author Humbart Santillo puts it, the superpowered protein molecules known as enzymes work in our bodies much the same way an electrical current illuminates a light bulb. Although the light bulb is in itself a wonderful physical structure, without electricity it is essentially lifeless. It simply cannot fulfill its purpose. Similarly, the human body cannot operate without the enzymes that fuel *all* our physical functions, including cell division, digestion, hormonal balance, immunity, mental acuity, metabolism, thyroid function, and even the absorption and assimilation of vitamins and minerals. In 1966, an article in a Scottish medical journal suggested that human beings and other living organisms could be defined as an "orderly, integrated succession of enzyme reactions." Without enzymes, we become lifeless.

A diet that is heavy in dairy products, meat, and cooked foods (vegan or otherwise) places stress on the body and can cause illness. It is imperative for true health that we consume a large percentage of enzyme-rich raw food and that we supplement with digestive enzymes. They play a critical role in the cleansing process.

tion, and just plain zip will help to fuel you, physically and mentally, through the 28 days of this program. Once the release of toxins has begun, your body is prepared to accept the next phase of the cleanse: rebuilding.

Rebuilding means weaning your properly prepared body back on the foods it was meant to rely on to keep it alive. It means revitalizing your cells, energizing your life processes, and, consequently, upgrading everything in your "physical plant," from your metabolism to your brain function to your ability to heal. As you begin to rebuild, I will give you the secrets I've accumulated over a quarter of a century to help you hasten your way back to optimal health. You'll learn, for example, which foods add nothing nutritionally and which may increase your susceptibility to disease. You'll discover how to read the signals your body sends and to give it the energy boosters it craves. Most of all, you'll learn to optimize the power of enzymes, which are, literally, the life force that vitalizes the foods we eat and our own bodies.

It is very clear to me now that what we put into our bodies does have a direct effect on our minds, hearts, and bodies. Open yourself up and miracles can occur! —**Anonymous**

Environmental Toxins

Of course, we all know that our planet has become increasingly polluted. Our systematic destruction of the rainforest and earth's other natural defenses has certainly been well documented. In this increasingly toxic world, we are exposed to damaging chemicals day and night, and often we don't even know it. For example, we jog on city streets, never considering that the air we're pulling into our lungs might counteract the benefits of exercise and even threaten our heart health. Then we quench our thirst with chemically treated water without giving a second thought to what it might be doing to our cells, our organs, or our bodies' miraculous physical systems.

More chemicals are making their way into the environment and into our bodies than ever before. According to the National Institute of Environmental Health Sciences, about 300 billion pounds of synthetic chemicals were produced, used, and disposed of in the United States in the early 1990s alone. Seventy years ago, that figure was closer to ten million pounds. All told, roughly eighty-four thousand chemicals are registered for commercial use in the United States.

So where are these chemicals right now? They are being pumped onto our neighbors' lawns, where they pollute the aquifer as runoff. They are in the clothes we bring home from the dry cleaners. They are incorporated into our shampoos, face creams, and other personal care products. They are in our household cleaners. They are even in our prescription drugs. And most worrisome, they are being absorbed through our skin and making their way through our digestive tracts.

Take a look around you right now. Think about your own surroundings and situation. Are you exposed to environmental pollutants like smog or secondhand smoke? Do you ingest alcohol, artificial sweeteners, caffeine, or food coloring? Are you aware that the foods you eat probably contain genetically modified organisms or growth hormones? Could these dangerous substances be setting you up for degenerative illness, obesity, premature aging, or worse? Are they the reason you're feeling so worn, so tired, so bloated, or just so lousy?

I know that thinking about the toxins that assault us in the course of normal, modern life is sobering and even frightening, but fear is not what I want to instill. Rather, I want you to become aware and to recognize that there is a solution to the problem. This solution is inherent in the natural instincts we are born with, even though we may have long forgotten.

WHY NATURE'S HEALING SYSTEM?

If you have ever browsed the shelves of a natural-food store, you have certainly seen the variety of cleansing systems available. Some are fiber-based products designed to move built-up toxins through the intestines. Others are liquid nutrition products that are used in conjunction with an herbal purgative. While there is no doubt that these products can help remove impurities from the digestive tract, in my experience they are superficial approaches. After all, you cannot expect to clear away toxins that have accumulated over a lifetime by using these products for just a few days.

These regimens do not properly prepare your body for maximum cleansing by providing you with delicious foods that cleanse as well as nourish. Nor do they help to rebuild the biological systems that keep you alive and healthy. These limited programs work like the cleansers we use on our kitchen floors. They strip off the top layer of old wax, but they don't make the room more efficient or a more inviting place in which to spend your time. With luck, you'll be spending a long time in the body that houses your spirit; it's important for you to be as comfortable in your skin as you can possibly be.

In comparison, my life-changing 28-day process works to rebalance your body, attuning it to the flavors and rhythms of nature. It doesn't matter if you begin this process as a hamburger-eating, cigar-smoking toxin collector. It doesn't matter if you have had a lifelong addiction to alcohol, animal fat, processed sugar, or anything else. Nature's Healing System will put you back in touch with your body's will to survive and thrive.

In 28 short days, you will break the bonds of self-destructive food cravings, even those that have haunted you throughout your life. You will learn to

use herbs to stop the sugar cravings that can undermine your health. You will discover the tasty, rewarding foods that optimize cleansing and burn fat while giving you a lasting feeling of fullness and satisfaction. You will end these transformative weeks with a new awareness of your health; a deeper connection with your body; and a more expansive, energetic consciousness.

A CHALLENGE

Give me four weeks and give yourself the gift of healing! It's this simple: 28 short days from now (or even sooner), you can wake up feeling better, looking better, and thinking more clearly about a future that suddenly seems brighter. Or you can spend the next four weeks eating and drinking the things that make your body a hospitable haven for aches, pains, chronic conditions, and, yes, even wrinkles and other signs of aging. Look in the mirror, get on the scale, review the results of your last medical checkup, and then read the dozens of unedited testimonials you'll find throughout this book. They are just a sampling of the thousands that have been shared with me. In the end, I believe you'll choose Nature's Healing System, which has been tested over time. I'm certainly not claiming that my program is the only way to detoxify—there are many roads to the top of the mountain—but I can claim that I have seen it work for thousands of people.

THREE RULES FOR A SUCCESSFUL CLEANSE

By this point, you are probably pretty excited to get started on this journey. Before you hit the ground running, let me emphasize three important rules that are essential to a successful detox. Over many years of teaching this program, I developed these rules for my students to help them avoid common pitfalls. Even though these rules may sound simple, many people find them hard to follow. I encourage you to keep coming back to these rules. You may even want to copy them down and post them where they can serve as a constant reminder.

RULE 1: For these 28 short days (and hopefully forever), make yourself number one. I know how difficult this can be, especially for the moms out there. There's always something to do—getting the kids to school, going to work, doing laun-

Nature's Healing System at a Glance

Chapters 2 through 4 will give you a breakdown of what you will do during each week of this cleansing program. You will engage in many healthful activities, including the following:

- aiding detoxification with body care
- cleansing internally with psyllium and detox clay
- drinking fresh vegetable and wheatgrass juices
- eating nutrient-dense raw vegan foods
- fasting for three days (liquids only)
- having colonics or enemas
- taking supplements and digestive enzymes

dry—that gets in the way of taking care of ourselves, even on the most basic level. Many of us, especially women, feel that we don't have the right to be self-centered, that taking care of ourselves and our health is selfish. But what good are you to yourself, your family, or your job if you are constantly feeling fatigued, stressed, and under the weather? I always remind people that I made my health the number one priority in my life, and that as a result I am able to help a lot of people. I am a better mother, grandmother, wife, and business owner because of it.

Don't put too much pressure on yourself in the beginning. Even if you need to read this book several times to absorb the information before you start detoxing, that's okay. Start making small changes so that healthful living becomes a greater part of your and your family's routine. You may not be able to do absolutely everything the first time around. The beauty is that the more you detox, the more energy you'll have. Just plan in advance and do the best you can. I recommend carving out a time for yourself each week to prepare everything you need in advance. Call it your healing day of preparation, even if it's only a few hours. Dedicate that short time to yourself and you'll be set up for success the rest of the week.

I thank you, Karyn, for saving me. You have no idea how much this [program] has helped me and changed my life. —S. J.

RULE 2: Don't judge yourself or others. For many of you, detoxing is a brand-new concept that may seem overwhelming. Just picking up this book is a huge step, let alone committing to this program and eating a mostly raw vegan diet for 28 days. Remind yourself that this journey is not about perfection. If you have a setback or are unable to do everything I recommend every single day, view it as an opportunity to learn, not as a failure. There is no judgment here—no good or bad, right or wrong. This is your own personal journey and a chance to get back in touch with your natural instincts, heal your body, and replenish your spirit.

You may not do the detox perfectly. You may give up after three days, or you may complete the program and have great results. But then life might get in the way and you won't make time for future cleanses. Whatever happens, at the very least try to read this book four times a year. Even if in the beginning you're munching on pepperoni pizza while doing so, you are planting seeds that will eventually grow into powerful ideas that you eventually won't be able to ignore. Think of it like advertising—no company airs a commercial once and expects you to run out and buy their product. They bombard you over and over through television, magazines, radio, and the Internet with ads and suggestive information until you finally believe you can't live

without whatever it is they're selling. It takes a long time for these messages to become programmed into your brain, and it will take time to replace them with new messages and beliefs. The key to my success has been surrounding myself with the information I share with you in this book—I read it, talk about it, and teach it every day to keep it programmed into my brain. Even if I slip up, I never judge myself. I blow kisses over each shoulder and remember that wherever I am and whatever I am doing is perfect. Give yourself a lot of credit. I certainly do!

RULE 3: Don't discuss what you are doing with others. As you begin your detox and start to experience the wonderful benefits of living in tune with nature, you are going to be tempted to share what you are doing with anyone and everyone who will listen. I encourage you not to, at least not until the end of Week 3. Even though your friends and family love you, they may not understand why you are drinking bottles of green liquid and not joining them for pizza and steak. If you need an excuse to get out of eating or drinking something that's not part of this program, tell people that you are on a special medication or you are getting tests done and you'll be back to "normal" soon. It's best not to let nay-saying and negative comments distract you during your cleanse.

If possible, find a cleansing buddy, such as a like-minded and open-minded friend, relative, or neighbor who is ready to go on this journey with you. That way, you can tap into the many benefits of the group experience that I witness in my classes. I find that people learn much more from each other than they do from me. I even discourage people from seeking private consultations with me because the group dynamic is so powerful. Sharing your progress, setbacks, miracles, and questions with a cleansing buddy will only enhance the journey.

However, if you absolutely can't find anyone to do the detox with you, confiding in trusted and nonjudgmental friends or relatives for support can be hugely beneficial. Just make sure they understand what you're doing and why, and that they are positive influences during your journey.

As a result of Karyn's detox program, I have felt magnificent every day! My energy level stays consistent (no midafternoon slumps), my skin is phenomenal, my hair has thickened, I've lost weight and toned up, my ability to focus on details has sharpened, my flexibility has increased greatly (I notice it most in my yoga practice), my eyes are whiter, and my mood has improved. I thought I was ahead of the game since I am vegan and exercise regularly, but this has shown me what I've been missing. —K. M.

I truly love doing this detox—it is such a rewarding experience. My skin has cleared up, I lost 20 pounds, and I have been able to balance my life emotionally. —M. F.

Thank you, Karyn, for helping me get in touch with my body. I wonder if the reason we end up with so many insecurities and health problems is because we just don't have a clue what our bodies want and need. —T. B.

I have had a sugar monkey on my back for as long as I can remember. Eventually it turned into hyperglycemia. Since the detox, I no longer think about trying to "get my fix" for most of the day like I used to, and this is a huge relief. —G.

Through the detox class I was able to deepen my knowledge of what my body needs. I feel more deliberate and mindful about what I put into my body and what I expose myself to. I am grateful to Karyn for jump-starting my path to self-healing. —E. K.

choices

DAYS 1 TO 7

We have all heard the saying "the journey is the destination." Day by day, moment by moment, life offers us choices. And these choices build upon each other, giving us direction, dimension, and character. It is as though we are each given a map and an innate sense of our ultimate destination. If we consciously choose our routes, if we go where we are supposed to go, either with or against traffic, we will eventually arrive at the appointed place. But if we do not choose, if we simply "go with the flow,"

we will end up wherever the flow happens to take us, whether that's where we want to be or not. In terms of your health and well-being, where has the flow taken you? Week 1 of the cleanse is about evaluating the choices we make and how they transform us, for better or for worse.

In our culture, where youth is currency, aging and health problems have given the publishing industry new life. Our degenerative diseases, fuzzy thinking, heartburn, indigestion, lack of libido, menopausal symptoms, overweight kids, wrinkles, and increasingly common chronic conditions have launched thousands of magazine articles, books, and even television sitcoms. Although some of the people behind this information explosion may mean well, the bottom line is that the media conditions us to believe that aging means illness, that every candle on the cake takes us further into the era of snuffed-out vitality, and that "life's a bitch and then you die"—but only after a prolonged and debilitating illness. Commercial interests profit from this kind of

I am a business owner, mother of two small children, wife, and active woman. I wanted to detox to prolong the quality of my life, learn an alternative way to eat, stop my migraines, and lose weight. In weeks, I have achieved my goals. I have not had one migraine headache. I have learned a wealth of information. I've lost 16 pounds. And my skin is so very soft and smooth. Thank you, Karyn, for adding longevity to my life and prosperity to my business. —L. T.

thinking. Did you ever notice the prevalence of prescription medication ads in some of our most popular "health" magazines?

How conditioned are your beliefs? When another birthday rolls around, do you think that, simply because the earth has spun on its axis one more time, you should look older? Feel older? Act older? Do you tell yourself that you have no control because, hey, who has control over the rotation of the planet? What do you tell your friends when they bemoan their own changes? Maybe "What do you expect? You aren't getting any younger," or "You have to face it—you're not twenty anymore." In a million ways, we tell ourselves and our friends that the cosmic alarm clock has ticked itself out. We say, "I can't wear that. I'm too old." Or perhaps we just issue a blanket statement like, "I'm older and that's that." It isn't long before messages like these become our mantras, our litanies, the internal tape loops that limit our thinking, negate our hopes, and lead us to physical debilitation.

By now, you might be feeling a little silly for accepting media messages about aging and the inevitable illness that comes with it. You shouldn't. The pharmaceutical industry, the dairy industry, producers of processed foods, and countless other businesses are built on our acceptance of the idea that aging comes with a lot of symptoms. If you're tired today, your joints ache, or you're gaining weight; if you have allergies, a sluggish metabolism, or skin problems; or if you're suffering from a laundry list of other minor and not-so-minor complaints, the most lucrative thing you can do about it, as far as American business is concerned, is to assume that you have no control over your symptoms.

Companies that do not have your best interests at heart earn megabucks when you believe that, no matter how lousy you feel, you can still eat all the french fries and ice cream and processed foods you want and wash them down with all the beer or fizzy aspartame you can drink. Don't let them convince you that your health has nothing to do with your habits. You have to keep your own best interests at heart. That means listening to your own body, not to the ads in magazines, in newspapers, and on television. No matter what the media would have you believe, you can get up every morning free from aches and pains and full of energy. Whatever your age, you don't have to be depressed, headachy, lethargic, or even forgetful. You don't have to become the next dialysis patient or cancer statistic. Rather, you have a choice. Whether you are entering menopause or living with chronic illness or even

Week 1 at a Glance

Begin the following:

- chlorella tablets
- digestive enzymes
- fenugreek seed capsules
- gentle exercise and bodywork
- Green Meal Shake
- journaling
- kamut water
- psyllium and detox clay
- rejuvelac
- vegan diet (no dairy, eggs, or meat)

For a detailed summary of the Week 1 cleansing protocol, see page 41.

trying to avoid the flu that is going around, you can be in total control of your health and well-being. I can promise you this because I am over sixty years old and I have not been sick in more than thirty years. I have made the choice to give my body what it needs to be healthy and vital. And you can too.

EATING LIVE TO STAY ALIVE

In our culture people closely associate with their ages. Based on the number of years I've been on this earth, most people would say that I am a middle-aged woman. That is not the way I describe myself, though. According to Gabriel Cousens, a physician who trained at the University of Chicago, the human body doesn't have a "use by" date that expires seventy-some years after birth. Human beings can live much longer, more vital lives, especially if they live far from the toxic culture that we call "civilization." Cousens believes that he has come in contact with a remote tribe in Greece where members claim to routinely live for over two hundred years! Can I prove to you that this is true? No. But the point is that we need to stop identifying ourselves with a number, stop believing that once we hit a certain age we are on a downward spiral and lose all control over our health and well-being.

A substantiated example is Okinawa, Japan, where a family-register system has recorded reliable birth, marriage, and death statistics since 1879. This information helps to identify centenarians, inhabitants who live beyond age one hundred. In Okinawa, there are thirty-four centenarians per hundred thousand inhabitants versus fewer than ten per hundred thousand in the United States. And many of them are healthy and active even at the end of life.

What about you? Is it reasonable for you to believe that you are over-the-hill? Or would you prefer, at age thirty or fifty or seventy, to think that you are still not within sight of the horizon? You may suspect that you have little in common with people who live on a Japanese island, but think about this: human bodies, wherever they are, have the same systems and basically operate the same way. Most of the body's cells and tissues renew themselves constantly, so that whatever your age, part of your body may be years younger. In fact, some scientists believe that most of our cells and tissues are never more than seven to ten years old. The difference between us and traditional Okinawan residents is that their diets and lifestyles encourage their cells to reproduce and replace themselves the way nature intended, while our lifestyles keep us from getting the oxygen and nutrition we need to do the same. Instead, we stuff ourselves with processed convenience foods that enable us to eat fast and die young.

The conditions that result from eating the standard American high-fat, nutrient-poor diet can seem inescapable, especially if you are already overweight

or suffering from arthritis, degenerative diseases, digestive problems, menopause symptoms, or other signs of premature aging. But the good news is that when we give the body what it needs to repair itself, it will. But I'm not the one who will prove that to you. In the next 28 days, you will prove it to yourself.

Don't get me wrong. I expect you to make healthful choices, but you can't go from A to Z overnight. You can't simply read a book and announce, "Eureka! I see the light! I'm going to give up alcohol, chocolate, cigarettes, meat, or whatever, and then my life will be perfect." In no endeavor do we expect to read about something and suddenly become an expert. We don't read a book about running and run a marathon the next day, or read a book about math and suddenly become mathematicians. Like everything in life, living in true health takes practice and dedication. The best way to transform your health and lifestyle over time is by detoxing your body regularly. I believe four times a year is ideal. At the very least, read this book and as much other information about natural health as you can. The more you expose yourself to this knowledge, the faster you will turn your symptoms and conditions around and achieve the best health of your life.

I had a slight weight problem, bad eating habits, and an addiction to diet tea. Then I met Karyn. I walked into her restaurant and standing before me was a forty-nine-year-old grandmother who looked twenty-two. She explained to me that she had been living a raw-food lifestyle for twenty-five years. That, along with a sampling of her food, changed my life. —S. B.

Cleansing your body of accumulated toxins is like peeling away the layers of an onion. Each time you detox, you reach a new strata of your being. As the poisons you have collected are released, their passing can affect you in unique and different ways. Each cleanse becomes an entirely distinct experience from the cleanse before.

To me and many of my clients, each 28-day detox is a reminder that, although we can't control the pollution and chemicals in our environments, we can control the chemicals we put into our mouths. As we begin to shed toxins and weight, we begin to get a clearer understanding of what our bodies were meant to be. Each cleanse becomes a map that shows us not only where we are right now in terms of our health, but also where we want to be and how to get there. With each subsequent cleanse, the route becomes clearer and clearer.

By now you are beginning to see the difference between what is considered "normal" in this culture and what is right and natural for the human body. Here is what is considered normal: mistaking the absence of diagnosed disease for health; eating greasy fast food instead of the healthful, natural foods that were meant to be our fuel; and prematurely sputtering out along life's highway. I propose that we forget the supposed normal for the next 28 days.

Instead, pay attention to what your body shows you during and after your detox. Your body is the authority. Although I am your guide through this transformational

journey, this cleanse is not about me. It is not even about you becoming a vegetarian or a vegan or a raw foodist, even if you believe these diets to be more healthful than your current way of eating. I can't tell you how many people have come up to me and said, "You know, Karyn, I'd love to do your program, but I just can't give up meat or cooked food or my glass of wine." I tell them that cleansing isn't about "giving up"; it's about "getting up" and starting out on your personal journey to your best possible self. The next thing I know, they've signed up for my detox class.

If you are like most of my clients, you have been on dozens of diets or nutritional regimens. You've tried all kinds of supplements and therapies in search of a magic bullet to cure what ails you. Although many diets or supplements have some value and are effective for temporary weight loss, I am willing to bet that none have truly made you come alive. I can promise you that in the next 28 short days, you will cast aside a lifetime of addictions. You will stop unconscious eating and start nourishing yourself. You will do things that you have never dreamed of and come to know your body as the miraculous, self-sustaining system it was meant to be. Most of all, you will be transformed, both physically and mentally, in a way that will enhance your life forever. Given this opportunity, I know you will choose to feed your body, renew your soul, and feel your best. Your joyful journey begins now, on Days 1 through 7.

WEEK 1: GO VEGAN

This chapter focuses on the first week of the cleanse, when the top priority is to eliminate unhealthful foods and replace them with nutrient-dense foods. By now it is obvious where we are headed: we are becoming vegans for the duration of this cleanse. This is your time to heal from the inside out. Healing is only possible when we stop ingesting the toxins that prevent our bodies from functioning the way nature intended. Following is information about the unfriendly foods I ask you to eliminate from your diet during Week 1.

Milk and Other Dairy Products

Got milk? If you have developed a tendency to gain weight or an inability to lose, if your sinuses are chronically congested, if you are prone to inexplicable symptoms like acne, constipation, headaches, indigestion, and rashes, then you probably consume milk and dairy products regularly. This shouldn't be a concern, should it? After all, we've been told that milk is the perfect food. In fact, it is—but only if you are a baby calf. Cow's milk is designed to do one thing: nourish a growing animal that packs on a whopping 800 pounds in the first year of its life.

For people, milk may be the most damaging food of all. Nature never intended human beings—or any species—to ingest the milk of another species.

Nearly every medical research group agrees that what Americans have come to regard as standard servings of meat are, in fact, dangerous amounts. We have the high cholesterol and blood pressure rates to prove it. Imagine my surprise, then, when a client with colon cancer presented me with the diet recommended for him by a very well-respected hospital. He was instructed to eat a high-protein diet with increased portions of meat, despite the proven link between animal fats and colon cancer. Why would medical professionals at a well-regarded institution make such a suggestion? Because feeding cancer patients a high-fat diet fattens them up so they don't look sick. I believe that eating meat is a good way to make you sick as well as fat.

Carnivorous animals were meant to eat meat. They are designed to digest and eliminate it very quickly. That's not the case with human beings. When we eat meat, it stays in our intestines for hours—typically thirty to thirty-five hours. We have come to accept this as normal, believing that stick-to-your-ribs food takes time to digest. But are your ribs what that steak dinner is sticking to? Think about it. Your intestines are hot, dark, and a constant 98 degrees Fahrenheit. What would happen if you took a steak, put it in a pipe, and laid it on the sidewalk on a 98-degree day? The steak would putrefy and rot, and quickly.

We may call it "meat," but make no mistake—the dyed, hormone-tainted cuts we find pristinely wrapped at the butcher's counter are simply packages of dead flesh and blood. What you cannot see through the plastic wrap are the steroids and antibiotics, routinely given to cows, that are now harbored in the meat. Meats are also tainted with the adrenaline, and hormones that surge through the cows before they are butchered. Anxious from days in transit and hours in crowded holding pens, the animals are forced into slaughterhouses, where the smell of death is all around them. They panic, just like we would under such duress. And just like us, they release a flood of hormones that are triggered by their fear. When we eat the flesh of these cattle, we literally ingest their terror. Is it any wonder that beef has been linked to so many chronic, degenerative, and fatal diseases?

Although chicken and fish may be marketed as healthful foods for weight loss, both are, in fact, loaded with saturated fat. Chicken has nearly as much cholesterol as beef, and make no mistake: eating it can increase your risk for heart disease. Eating fatty fish increases total and saturated fat intake and can result in higher cholesterol levels and weight gain. Just like their bovine counterparts, commercially farmed chicken and fish are given antibiotics to combat their toxic environments and hormones to make them larger and therefore more profitable.

I have found from my own experience that chicken is a dangerously contaminated food. When I first opened a restaurant, I took a course offered by the health department to learn about safe food preparation and cleanliness standards. I learned then, some twenty years ago, that chicken had to be heated to 140 degrees Fahrenheit to kill all salmonella in the flesh. Ten years later, that temperature went up to 160 degrees, and now, only twenty years later, chickens have become so susceptible to disease that health officials have raised the required cooking temperature to 175 degrees Fahrenheit. It is also required by law that chickens be stored only on the bottom shelf of a commercial refrigerator. The slightest contact with chicken drippings is considered contamination. Any food that is contaminated by exposure to chicken juices can cause severe illness or even death.

Because the earth's water supply is now so polluted, fish and shellfish constantly absorb dangerous contaminants, including chemical compounds, pesticides, and heavy metals. Nearly all fish and shellfish contain traces of mercury. Many people are aware that pregnant women should avoid eating mercury-tainted fish because it can damage their children's nervous systems. The U.S. Food and Drug Administration and the Environmental Protection Agency recommend that women who are pregnant avoid or limit eating certain types of fish, including albacore tuna, shark, swordfish, king mackerel, and tilefish. People who have compromised immune systems should also be especially careful to avoid mercury poisoning. The bottom line is that mercury is a dangerous toxin for everyone because it damages the cardiovascular and central nervous systems. In addition, mercury is a known human carcinogen.

After your cleanse, you may decide to return to eating animal products. However, like many of my clients, you may be more scrupulous about the kinds of animal products you eat. For example, you may switch to buying organic. Note, however, that even organic or free-range options are not necessarily safe substitutes for factory-farmed animal foods. For now, see for yourself whether like begets like—whether you look and feel more alive eating living, vital foods than the flesh of dead animals. Your transformation will astound you.

The information I've given you up to this point may motivate you to eschew dairy products, eggs, meat, chicken, and fish forever. However, right now I don't want you to focus on forever or on making sweeping declarations. Rather, I want you to mentally sign up for this journey one week at a time, if not one day at a time. The quickest way to fall off the wagon is to commit to too much at once. As I always say, make it practical to keep it in practice.

WEEK 1: WHAT YOU CAN HAVE

Now that I've told you everything I'm asking you not to eat this week, let's talk about the wonderful healing foods and supplements that you *can* have. For many people who are new to the cleanse, their greatest concern is what they will be eating for the next 28 days. That's because many of the foods that are most convenient are the ones that are bad for you. (And yes, I do take exception to those people who insist there are no bad foods—there are!) Within the first hour of class, I announce to my detoxers that most of the foods they reach for automatically—the cheese, the roast beef sandwich, the ice cream cone, the extra-crispy fried chicken—are forbidden. That statement can leave them confused about their options.

For example, here is what one participant had to say: "What was I thinking during the first session of Karyn's cleanse? Halfway through, I wasn't thinking about my health. I wasn't even really thinking about what I wanted to change. To be honest, all I was thinking was, 'What in the world am I going to eat?'"

The truth is that during Days 1 through 7, you can choose from an extensive variety of delicious vegan specialties, including many dishes that you may already enjoy. Hummus, tabbouleh, vegetable stir-fries, vegetarian chili—virtually anything you can create using a good vegan cookbook is a perfectly acceptable, very satisfying way to ease into the detox. Search for vegan and vegetarian restaurants where you live; there are more and more these days. Almost any conventional restaurant you go to will have a vegetarian option, or the chef will be happy to prepare a dish for you on request. Lucky for us, veganism is now much more popular than it was even a few years ago.

Whatever your current approach to eating, remember that the first week of the cleanse is about choices. I think you'll find that the foods and supplements I suggest for Days 1 through 7 will empower you to make the best possible choices—for the cleanse, for your health, and for your longevity.

Find Supplements Online

Beyond eating vegan foods, you'll be adding a variety of supplements during your first week of the cleanse. Some of these may be unfamiliar to you. If you're worried about where to purchase these items, many are available on my website, www.karynraw.com, or from a reputable natural-food store. Just be certain to make sure that all the items you purchase are vegan.

Green Meal Shake (page 108)

Although it is the color of the front lawn, this delicious meal in a glass is the most popular raw food that detoxers carry into their postcleanse lives. This powerful, detoxifying smoothie really does have it all: the natural sweetness of apple juice and banana, the protective omega-3 fatty acids of flaxseed oil, and the B vitamins

and probiotics of rejuvelac (see the next section and the recipe on page 106). The Green Meal Shake also contains lecithin, a natural thickener that makes it creamy and delicious. As a bonus, lecithin also is great for your brain and arteries.

The main ingredient in the Green Meal Shake is my Karyn's Kare Green Meal Powder. Many years ago I customized this blend of sprouted grains, grasses, and sea vegetables to provide a healthful dose of calcium, minerals, proteins, vitamins, and much more. Starting your day with a smoothie made from this superfood powder is a great way to have a complete, filling, and alkalizing raw meal. The Green Meal Shake will feed your body and satisfy your need for fats, creamy texture, and a sweet taste. Most people are completely satisfied for three to five hours after drinking a Green Meal Shake. If your budget allows, use organic fruit. Otherwise, toss in the best ingredients you can afford. If you don't use my smoothie powder, please make sure you are substituting with a vegan, plant-based product that is free from fillers and protein isolates.

For those of you who are put off by the color of this wonderful drink, think about this: we have become programmed to enjoy fake colors and flavors that are formulated in laboratories, not in nature. Given the chance, you may find you have the same powerful attraction to the colors of nature. Many clients have told me that this shake keeps them from the cookie jar in times of stress. Mix enough for a few days at once (and store it in glass jars in the refrigerator) so that this ultimate convenience food is always within reach when hunger strikes. Try it for three days and you'll be hooked.

WEEK 1: Begin drinking one Green Meal Shake every day. You can drink the shake anytime, but my clients typically choose to have it as the first meal of the day.

Rejuvelac (page 106)

At the onset of the cleanse, people either love this deeply healing fermented drink or they hate it. Nevertheless, rejuvelac is so nourishing, so curative, and so incredibly satisfying that by Week 2, virtually everybody begins to crave it. Rejuvelac is easy to make, but it can also be purchased at some natural-food stores, including my own.

Rejuvelac was developed by Dr. Wigmore and is a vitamin-rich, nutritional powerhouse. It is physically rejuvenating ("rejuv") and rich in lacto bacteria ("lac"). But don't think that it's made with milk because of the term "lacto." Rejuvelac is made by sprouting wheat berries and then soaking the sprouted wheat berries in purified

I deliberately did not weigh myself before the start of the program. I wasn't interested in what was on the scale. My heartfelt desire was to begin a true health quest. With this program, I believe I have all the tools needed to begin taking control of my health. I enjoyed the rejuvelac—and most of all, I am happy to report that I have not craved any sweets. —D. H.

water. Left at room temperature to ferment for several days, the soaking water becomes an enzymatically alive liquid that is rich in the beneficial bacteria lactoba-cillus. Fermented foods are an important part of raw and living-food diets.

In fact, rejuvelac is such an energizing, purifying drink, it won't be long before you start to wonder how you ever lived without it. Fermented foods and drinks like rejuvelac are key to a balanced internal ecology. The nondairy lactobacil-lus not only destroys harmful bacteria in the intestines, it also establishes benefi-cial bacteria that strengthen immunity, aid digestion, reduce candida growth, and cleanse the intestinal tract. Sprouted wheat berries are brimming with B vitamins, which, in addition to being essential nutrients, soothe the effects of stress through-out the body. Moreover, each sip of rejuvelac provides you with digestible protein and a vitalizing, oxygenated food. I like to call this profoundly nutritious living food "the nutrition ignition of the health conscious."

WEEK 1: Begin drinking two or three 8-ounce glasses of rejuvelac each day. This includes the glass you blend into your Green Meal Shake.

Digestive Enzymes

Supplementation with digestive enzymes is one of the most effective ways to support your digestive process. The digestive process is the hardest working sys-tem in our body, and most of us really put it to task. In her book *The Healing Power of Enzymes*, DicQie Fuller writes, "Eighty percent of our body's energy is expended by the digestive process. If you are run down, under stress, living in a very hot or very cold climate, pregnant, or a frequent traveler, then enormous quantities of extra enzymes are required by your body. Aging deprives us of our ability to produce necessary enzymes."

A lack of digestive enzymes can lead to allergies, constipation, gas, heart-burn, and a host of other problems. As you age, you may find you are not able to tolerate certain foods anymore. Ever wonder why people develop allergies and become lactose or gluten intolerant later in life? Enzyme supplementation preserves your vitality by assisting during the early stages of digestion, lightening the load on the pancreas later in the process.

I developed Karyn's Kare Digestive Enzymes with my teacher and a true enzyme expert, Viktoras Kulvinskas. If you choose not to take my enzymes, however, make sure you choose a brand that is plant-based. Not only are plant-based enzymes free of animal products, they are also better equipped to survive in a wider pH range, making them more effective in acidic environments (like your stomach).

On a 99.9 percent raw diet, I still take about twenty digestive enzymes a day. If that sounds like a lot to you, rest assured that there has never been an enzyme

overdose reported. However, if you develop stomach cramps or diarrhea, cut back on the number you are taking.

WEEK 1: Begin taking digestive enzymes with every meal. Take a minimum of three digestive enzymes before any meal or snack, but you can take many more than that.

Green Kamut Powder

Kamut is an ancient grain, considered an heirloom grain because it has remained unchanged and unhybridized throughout history. Archeologists even found kamut in King Tut's tomb. The Karyn's Kare Green Kamut Powder that we use during the cleanse is a blend of dehydrated wheatgrass juice and healing aloe vera. Like the Green Meal Shake (page 108), the color of kamut water may scare you at first. However, this chlorophyll-rich drink will not only quench your thirst, it will also draw poisons from your body, build up your blood, and repair your white blood cells.

WEEK 1: Begin drinking kamut water every day. Add 1 to 2 tablespoons of Green Kamut Powder to 16 ounces of water and sip it throughout the day. Because green kamut is a very light powder, you will find it easier to mix in a blender rather than with a spoon. Kamut water can be made ahead of time, poured into glass jars, and stored in the refrigerator for up to five days.

Chlorella Tablets

Chlorella is an algae and another chlorophyll-rich food. Chlorella cleanses the gastrointestinal (GI) tract and strengthens the peristaltic muscles of the colon, which propel digesting material through your system. It is a powerful tool for healing digestive issues.

WEEK 1: Begin to chew six chlorella tablets twice a day. You can take them anytime, with food or on an empty stomach. I must warn you that chlorella will momentarily coat your teeth green and may even get stuck between them. It's worth the temporary unsightliness, however. Just make sure you check the mirror before carrying on a conversation.

Fenugreek Seed Capsules

You have probably noticed that I haven't suggested that you remove sugar from your diet. I've observed that when people abruptly stop eating animal products, they might start craving sugar. Now, a bit of natural sugar is not a bad thing. You can

Symptoms Are Messages

As you already know, I am not a fan of unnecessary medication or a proponent of the magic little pill. Through the media—and our doctors—we get the idea that when something ails us, we need only take some amazing new chemical compound and our problems will be solved. Of course, I'm not telling you not to take medication. I'm simply reminding you that our symptoms are messages from our bodies to let us know something's wrong.

If you are driving your car, for instance, and the brake light comes on, you wouldn't just get out, snip the wire, and keep driving, or you'd be headed for disaster. Medications can be like that. They usually don't eliminate a disorder. Instead, they simply eradicate the error message. If you have a headache and take an aspirin, the headache may go away. However, that doesn't mean that you had a headache because your body was lacking an aspirin. Rather, you had a headache because there was an underlying problem that you haven't addressed.

make many easy and delicious raw desserts using agave nectar, dates, stevia, or any natural sweetener you prefer. Nevertheless, one of your goals during the cleanse is to get your body in balance. In order to accomplish that, it is best to cut down on sugar. Fenugreek seed capsules can help.

Fenugreek is an herb that has been used medicinally and in cooking by Asian and Mediterranean people since ancient times. A potent, herbal remedy, fenugreek has earned a reputation as a detoxifier and blood builder. It is also very helpful in combating one of the most rampant addictions created by the food industry—that is, America's endless hunger for sugar. Lucky for me and all detoxers, fenugreek seed banishes sugar cravings. In fact, a few days into the cleanse, you may find that fenugreek works so well, the desserts you love may start tasting *too* sweet. Many of my clients claim that this simple herb can banish a sweet tooth forever.

WEEK 1: Begin taking three fenugreek seed capsules twice a day. Just don't be surprised if you detect the distinct aroma of this herb around your underarms after a few days. Fenugreek helps to dissolve hardened masses of accumulated mucus, and it also helps to expel toxins from the body through the lymphatic system. Since many of your lymph nodes are located under your arms, the fenugreek scent will remind you that your body is reacting to the cleanse and beginning to rebalance itself.

Psyllium and Detox clay

There is no true cleansing without removing mucus, hardened wastes, and impurities from the colon. Fiber promotes colonic activity, and psyllium seed is an excellent source. The addition of psyllium and detox clay to your cleansing regimen will ensure that the toxic residues that cause disease, discomfort, and premature aging are expelled every day of your 28-day program.

The research is irrefutable. By simply increasing our daily intake of fiber, we can reduce our risk of diabetes, digestive disorders, heart attack, obesity, stroke, and a host of degenerative diseases. Psyllium powder, made from the dried husks of the psyllium seed, is a gentle, natural product that speeds the movement of mucus from the body while providing an adequate dose of fiber to help get your bowels

moving. Detox clay, a powder made from volcanic ash, pulls the impurities from the deep crevices of your colon. I sell a detox clay powder, but you may find it in liquid form, which is perfectly acceptable. Just make sure it is a pure clay with no added fillers.

I admit, psyllium and detox clay may be less palatable than anything else you will consume during this cleanse. Psyllium's gelatinous texture takes some getting used to, and detox clay definitely tastes like the ash that it is. Nevertheless, these two important products, used in conjunction, will speed the passage of toxins out of your body like nothing else. You will begin to have wonderful bowel movements (BMs) so worthy of note that you may find yourself discussing them with your cleansing buddy or anyone who's willing to listen.

Here's an amusing example. A man who was in one of my classes was on his way to a wedding with his girlfriend. Dressed in his tux, he dropped by my restaurant and found me by the juice bar. He said, "I just wanted you to know that what you said was true. My BMs are absolutely incredible!" I asked him whether he ever thought he would one day walk into a restaurant wearing a tuxedo to brag about his bowel movements. It may seem like an improbable tale but, after a few days of the psyllium and detox clay, don't be surprised if you find yourself doing something like this too.

WEEK 1: Begin drinking your psyllium-detox clay cocktail every day. If you have normal bowel movements and evacuate every day or more than once a day, I recommend that you take 1 tablespoon each of psyllium and detox clay in the evening. If you suffer from constipation and evacuate only every other day or, as I used to do, once a week (incredibly, the doctors told my mother it was just my system!), use 1 teaspoon of psyllium and 1 tablespoon of detox clay in the evening. While you might think that people with sluggish bowels would benefit from an increased dosage, the opposite is true. Underactive bowels may cause the psyllium-detox clay mixture to clog the colon.

I have found that the best way to get the psyllium-detox clay cocktail down is to add 1 tablespoon of detox clay and 6 ounces of water to a shaker cup. Shake the cup until it is combined. Then add the psyllium, shake three times, and chug. The longer you wait before consuming it, the thicker the mix will become and the harder it will be to get down. Immediately follow with 10 ounces of water.

Take psyllium and detox clay at least forty minutes before or after eating or taking any supplements. Ideally, take it before going to bed. Psyllium and detox clay are forces to

A Snack for Week 1

This snack is a great bridge for those who are moving from cooked to raw foods. Mix equal parts of Karyn's Lemon-Herb Dressing (page 115) and dulse, and spread the mixture on a slice of Manna bread. This brand of bread is cooked, but it is made from sprouted grains, making it an optimal choice. During the cleanse I only recommend the millet variety of Manna bread.

be reckoned with. If you take them too close to a mealtime, they will draw nutrients from the food and move them through your intestines too quickly. So try to stave off your hunger until the psyllium and detox clay have done their work.

YOU HAVE THE POWER

No matter how far we take the process, no matter how far the process takes us, cleansing is a journey that transforms us from the inside out. The choices you make during Days 1 through 7 will direct your attention away from the external details of life—such as your responsibilities at work, your chores, your to-do list, or the opinions of others—and focus your understanding on the internal concerns that shape you physically, mentally, and spiritually.

You are likely to find the first week of the cleanse to be a truly consciousness-raising experience. For the first time perhaps in years, you will feel your body responding to what you eat and healing itself. You will sense your systems working the way they should, drawing energy from food. Gradually, you will become aware of a growing feeling of control over your eating patterns and your health. You may even begin to feel a profound appreciation for your body and an increased confidence that, whatever shape you're in, whatever your current physical challenges, you have the power to transform your future.

Gentle Exercise and Bodywork

During Week 1, focus more deeply on the changes in your body by beginning a program of gentle exercise. Meditative walks or spiritual yoga sessions will lead you to a deeper understanding of the body-mind connection that directs your behavior and health. Keep in mind that a true yoga practice is about the connection between the body and mind, not sweating yourself dry or getting in a challenging workout. Jumping on a mini trampoline will help your lymphatic system drain itself of accumulated toxins. In addition, you may opt to have a series of chiropractic adjustments to enhance the effects of the cleanse. Spinal adjustment can strengthen the relationship between the nervous system and the health of the whole body by releasing impinged spinal nerves. Practicing qigong or having a massage can also enhance your body's ability to heal itself as nature intended.

Journaling

Now is a great time to begin a cleansing journal. Try to commit your feelings and results to paper at least once a day so that you have a record of your experience. For example, you may write about what you've ingested on a given day and the

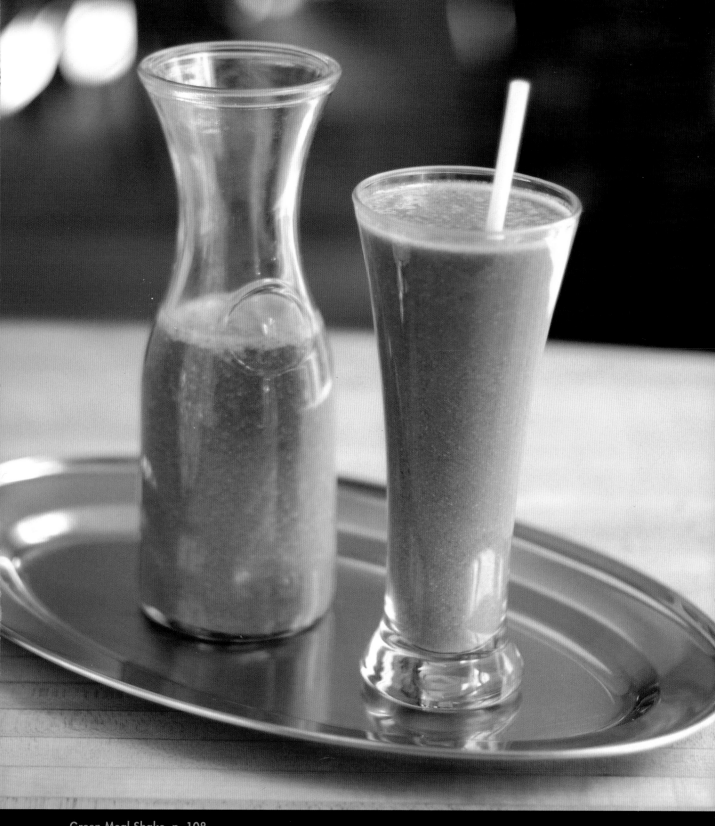

Green Meal Shake, p. 108

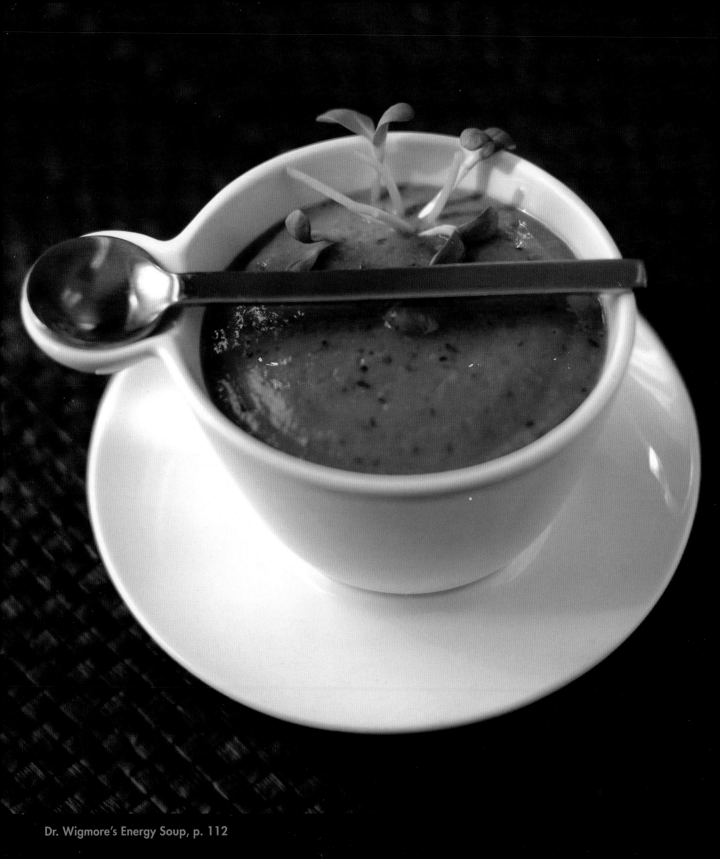

Dr. Wigmore's Energy Soup, p. 112

cleansing reactions that followed. Most importantly, your journal will provide you with an ongoing chronicle of your progress. Cleansing can be like watching grass grow; the day-to-day effects can be subtle. Even the changes that seem remarkable at the time, such as the onset of cleansing symptoms or the sudden disappearance of a minor chronic condition, can be overlooked like yesterday's news once you've adjusted to the change.

Your journal will remind you of each stage of your transformation. Reviewing a previous entry may inspire you to persevere when your unhealthful addictions begin to fight back. Most of all, a record of the tips, techniques, and secrets that make your personal process easier can help pave the way for your next detox or even speed your cleansing process. Allow yourself time to commit all your observations to paper and your journal will become the one book you've always wished you had: the owner's manual to your body.

OPTIMIZING THE CLEANSE

If you begin to feel during the first week that you are ready to take the cleanse further, especially if you are an old hand at detoxing, you may begin your raw vegan diet during Week 1. Raw food will not only improve your digestion and cleanse your colon, it will also begin to oxygenate and alkalize your body. Starting a raw diet now may quicken the onset of cleansing symptoms, so be prepared. Just remember that the headache, chills, runny nose, or whatever physical "blessing" you receive is a sign that toxins are on their way out of your body. As they say, better out than in.

If you feel you might want to go raw during Week 1, stock up on raw snacks before you begin your cleanse. Try sprouting or experimenting with easy raw-food recipes. See a small sampling of recipes in chapter 6 (pages 106 to 116) and a list of raw-food recipe books in Resources (page 119). You may even want to try something that two of my busy clients did. They joined forces to set up a sprouting and food-preparation co-op. They agreed that they would each sprout different seeds so they would have an interesting array to share. They also agreed to make double batches of the recipes they wanted to try. As a result, they always had an interesting raw dinner entrée at the ready. They were never hungry and never felt deprived. Best of all, when their families sat down at the table to eat and socialize, they did too.

During Week 1, read the next chapter of this book. It will prepare you in every way to go raw. When you do, listen to your body's cues and don't worry about the amount of food you're eating. With every mouthful, you are literally taking in the life force that will renew you. As you reacquaint yourself with your body, you will learn to recognize when you need to eat and when you've eaten enough.

A FINAL WORD

Aclient who was in the middle of her cleanse related the reaction of a friend she met one day at the local market. When the woman asked her out for a quick bite, my client briefly described the cleansing program.

"Let me get this straight," the friend gasped. "You can't eat dairy or meat or chicken. You can't even eat fish! So what on earth can you eat?"

Virtually everyone who tries my program spends a good deal of time thinking about the foods they will eliminate for 28 days. For them, cheese, eggs, and hamburgers are habits. Nutritious or not, these are the foods that most people eat and find satisfying. But are we really satisfied by these foods? Are satisfied people subject to food cravings? Is constantly searching through the refrigerator for the next snack or the next meal a sign of someone who has eaten something that satisfies his or her metabolic needs? I think not.

Rather than focus on what you will not be eating during Week 1, consider the delicious, exciting variety of foods available to you. Your body knows what is good for it. Your body wants to survive. If you give your body what it is supposed to have, the fuel that enables it to thrive, I guarantee that your cravings will disappear just as mine have.

For now, I suggest that you separate yourself from people whose negative comments and off-the-cuff criticism might undermine your success. Most of us have already sacrificed enough in our effort to win the approval of people who don't necessarily have our best interests at heart.

If you're feeling guilty about consciously avoiding some of your nearest and dearest now, I'll guarantee that in a couple of weeks they'll be beating down your door to ask whether you've lost weight, why you look so rested, or where you got that healthy glow. Go ahead and invite them in for a green drink (or a raw dessert). When they see the new you, they may be more than willing to try a cleanse too.

WEEK 1: FREQUENTLY ASKED QUESTIONS

Q: What kind of water do you recommend?

A: I alternate between distilled water and alkalized or ionized water. Your choice may depend on how much you're prepared to spend. There are a host of sophisticated water systems to choose from, but any filtered water is fine. Even using a Brita water filter or another inexpensive filtration system is great. I just encourage you not to use water directly from the tap.

Q: I noticed that the dosages you recommend for each product are different from what appears on the product bottles. Why is that?

A: Remember that during detox we are in boot camp. We are taking in as much healing chlorophyll as possible, and we are primed and ready for any symptoms that may arise. After the detox is over, you are welcome to follow the bottle instructions for any products you choose to continue. However, like most of my clients, you will probably find that the detox dosages are more your speed.

Q: Are wheat products allowed during Week 1 of the cleanse?

A: Wheat products are allowed during Week 1; however, they are not optimal. If you must have bread, I recommend Manna or Essene brands, which are available in the freezer section of most natural-food stores. Although these breads are cooked, the grains are soaked and sprouted first and then heated to much lower temperatures than most breads. Therefore, they retain more nutrients and are easier to digest. After Week 1, however, I ask that you limit yourself to raw dehydrated crackers or bread that you can find in my store and other natural-food stores. Just make sure that the package indicates that the crackers or bread are raw. It may be helpful to search for some trusted brands on the Internet before you go shopping. Or ask an employee for guidance when you are at the store.

Q: I am gluten intolerant. Can I have rejuvelac, kamut, and wheatgrass?

A: The gluten protein in wheat, oats, rye, and barley is fully activated in the cooking process. When a gluten grain is soaked and sprouted, the gluten protein may not be activated at all, making rejuvelac, kamut, and wheatgrass perfectly tolerable even for those with gluten sensitivities. I suggest that you test your tolerance very carefully and possibly under the care of your physician. Allergies and intolerances are often a result of excess mucus in the digestive tract. You may rid yourself of these sensitivities through regular cleansing, which will allow you to enjoy the healing power of rejuvelac, kamut, wheatgrass, and any other raw food containing wheat, oats, rye, and barley.

Q: You didn't mention coffee or alcohol. Can I still consume them?

A: I took a lot away from you during Week 1. If I didn't mention something, it's better not to ask! During this first week I am not officially taking away coffee and alcohol, but if you can give them up, all the better. I recommend that you drink an alkalizing beverage, like kamut water or the Green Meal Shake, before you have your coffee or alcohol, as they will help balance the acidity. In addition, as you bring your body into balance with chlorophyll-rich foods, you may find that your taste, need, and tolerance for coffee and alcohol diminish naturally.

Q: Is it possible to stay on this program while I'm traveling?

A: I travel for business and pleasure all the time and so do many of my clients. One client, a busy attorney, carries her supplies in zipper-lock plastic bags and

mixes her drinks in her hotel room. There's no place like the hotel minibar to store rejuvelac, kamut water, and premixed shakes. I also prepare as much as possible in advance and keep everything frozen until I arrive at my destination.

Q: I'm a little daunted by the prospect of going raw. Is there a way to ease into it?

A: Yes, you can ease into eating raw. There is no better time for it than during Week 1. While you are eating vegan, begin adding certain raw foods to your diet. Since convenience is the key to success for any eating program, make some raw snacks that are easy to grab when you walk in the door—dehydrated foods are your friends. Begin sprouting lentils or beans for salads or entrees. Try one new recipe a day so that by the end of the week you have a number of recipes in your repertoire. See a small sampling of recipes in chapter 6 (pages 106 to 116) and a list of raw-food recipe books in Resources (page 119). Once you get started, I think you'll find that raw foods aren't really so alien. They are the nourishment that was intended for us.

Q: I just counted the calories in the Green Meal Shake and was surprised to see that it is much higher in calories than my regular breakfast. Is it possible that I'll actually gain weight while detoxing?

A: Calories are far less important than the quality of the food you are ingesting. Your body will absorb vitamins and minerals from raw natural foods far more effectively than the foods that make up the standard American diet. The healthful fats founds in nature actually help your body burn fat. I encourage you to stop counting calories and worrying about the government's cookie-cutter guidelines or recommended daily values. Instead, start listening to your body's hunger cues and feed it the nutrient-rich foods that sustain and regenerate it.

Q: I'm having a problem with the texture of the psyllium and detox clay mixture. It's so thick. I just can't seem to get it down. Do you have any advice?

A: If you mix your psyllium and detox clay in very cold water, it won't congeal as rapidly. Then you can quickly drink it and follow with a glass of water immediately after. In an absolute pinch, you can even mix the psyllium and detox clay with applesauce and eat it with a spoon. Just bear in mind that we are working to stabilize your blood sugar levels, so turning this treatment into a dessert is not an optimal solution.

Q: I can't find some of the products you recommend at my natural-food store. Can I order them from you?

A: Absolutely! All the products I recommend can be purchased online at www.karynraw.com. For my additional contact information, see Resources, page 119.

TABLE 1. Week 1 protocol summary

Use these summaries to map out a plan prior to starting each week of the cleanse. Some of my clients measure every-thing out for their week in advance; others create checklists for themselves. Any planning you can do to organize your detox will help ensure you don't get overwhelmed during this wonderful healing process.

FOOD/PRODUCT	INSTRUCTIONS	TIMING	BENEFITS
Vegan diet	Avoid all animal products, including dairy, eggs, meat, chicken, and fish.	Pay attention to your body's cues and eat snacks or full meals when you are truly hungry.	Eating a cooked vegan diet during Week 1 will begin to clean out your system and prepare you for the raw diet to come in Weeks 2, 3, and 4. If you feel you can incorporate raw food into your Week 1 diet, all the better.
Green Meal Shake	Have one Green Meal Shake each day. The recipe on page 108 makes 1 (16-ounce) shake.	Drink as the first meal of the day or anytime during the day.	The Green Meal Shake is a nutrient-dense raw superfood that is easy for your body to digest. It improves metabolism and calcium absorption.
Rejuvelac	Drink 2 or 3 (8-ounce) glasses of rejuvelac, or as much as you like, each day.	Sip throughout the day. Use as an ingredi-ent in your Green Meal Shake.	Rejuvelac is good for stress and helps clean the intestinal tract by loosening mucus. It contains B vitamins, enzymes, and protein. It is a nondairy source of the beneficial bacteria lactobacillus.
Digestive enzymes	Take with all meals. For weight loss, take 4 to 5 capsules before eating, 3 to 4 capsules during your meal, and 2 capsules after eating.	Take before, during, and after each meal.	Digestive enzymes break down food so that nu-trients quickly pass through the intestinal walls, circulate through the bloodstream, and nourish the body's cells.
Kamut water	Mix 2 tablespoons of Green Kamut Powder in 16 ounces of purified water. If possible, mix kamut water in a blender. Pulse or mix on slow speed.	Sip throughout the day.	Kamut draws out poisons and builds up the blood by repairing the white blood cells. It also stimulates energy.
Chlorella tablets	Take 6 tablets, 2 times a day. Chew the tablets thoroughly. Do not swallow them whole.	Take anytime during the day.	Chlorella strengthens the peristaltic muscles in the colon, improving digestion and elimination, and is especially effective in treating lower GI issues. It helps the body to remove heavy metals and environmental toxins.
Fenugreek seed capsules	Take 3 capsules 2 times a day.	Take in the morning and early evening.	Fenugreek loosens and expels mucus, dead waste matter, and toxins through the lymphatic system. It also balances blood sugar levels.
Psyllium-detox clay cocktail	Mix 1 teaspoon or tablespoon (use the lesser amount if you have slow bowels or are con-stipated) of psyllium and 2 tablespoon of detox clay in 4 to 6 ounces of purified water. Cover, shake 3 times, and drink. Follow with 10 ounces of purified water.	Take last thing at night. Wait at least 40 minutes after eating or drinking other foods.	The psyllium-detox clay cocktail cleanses mucus-forming toxic waste from the colon. The detox clay can also be used topically in a facial mask to draw toxins through the skin. (See page 98.)

SYMPTOMS OF CLEANSING

I've already mentioned the potential cleansing reactions you could experience during the detox, but I want to remind you once again that these healing crises are perfectly normal and should be welcomed. Nothing will derail you faster than worrying about each and every symptom that may arise. Remember that any condition you're already struggling with can get worse before it gets better. Of course, you must follow your instincts. If you feel a symptom has gotten out of your control, make a judgment call about what the right decision is for you, even if it means stopping the detox or scaling back on some of the protocol. This list contains some of the most common symptoms of cleansing. Refer to it every time a symptom arises and see if you can't power through it.

- acne
- bad breath
- body odor
- chills
- diarrhea
- dry eyes
- dry mouth
- fatigue
- fever
- flulike symptoms
- headaches
- nausea
- pain blockage
- rash
- runny nose/mucus drainage
- sore throat
- vomiting

I was always fatigued and sluggish. Being a mother with small children, I thought I owed it to myself and my kids to live a healthier life. I have more energy now, the swelling and pain in my feet are gone, my skin is clearer, and I've even lost weight. I'm sharing my stories with friends and family, hoping they'll take the journey too. —D. C.

The detox was a great experience. My favorite part was the surplus energy and happiness I felt (and continue to feel). I am thankful for the clarity I've experienced and for my greater consciousness about food. I have made a permanent life change. —C. O.

I love Karyn's approach because it is comprehensive and includes a strict cleansing regimen as well as a nutritional component, which is important for healing the diseased body and mind. —C. D.

My experience during detox has opened my eyes to the unlimited health possibilities attainable through food. I knew that my body was changing by the way my face looked and my clothes fit. I have obtained energy, calmness, and clarity. —J. H.

After discovering that I was chemically sensitive, I have been trying everything to regain my health. This amazing program provided inspiration, scientific research, and vital information that resonated with me. This was the last leg of a very long, very challenging journey. The knowledge Karyn has given me about how to live is priceless. —M. J. D.

My stomach is flat, my PMS symptoms are nonexistent, and my skin is hydrated. My goal was to get rid of the symptoms that I started with, and I was successful. —T. B.

I entered the class with high expectations that I did not believe would be met. I had no idea that the program could make such a dramatic difference, and I do mean dramatic! I have surpassed all my objectives. What I have been unable to do in four years, I did in one month. —C. M.

This wonderful process opened some very important new areas of life to me. Not only have there been obvious physical benefits, but my clarity of thought and spiritual connections have also taken on added dimensions. I was pleasantly surprised to discover my inner strength to stick with the program. —B. C.

Karyn's program is the only service or product I can recall being involved with that has done exactly what it said it would do and provided precisely the results promised—and with amazing effectiveness. —N. S.

I will be 40 soon, and my goal in attending the class was to begin "reinventing" myself as I embark on the second best half of my life. I have achieved many positive benefits: my skin is clearer, I have greater mental clarity, and my clothes fit much better too. With this program, I have all the tools I need to take control of my health. —D. H.

changes

D A Y S   8   T O   1 4

Virtually every adult I know has been on a diet. And virtually everyone who's been on a diet has had an experience like the following: It is Day 3 of your program. Your stomach feels so empty you think you hear an echo in your abdomen every time you speak. Nevertheless, you carefully continue to weigh and prepare each morsel of every meal. Day after day, you eat precisely what is specified by your plan—not a bite more or less. Then one morning a week or so into the diet, you awake with a

realization. Although you began this program to enhance your health, you feel just as sluggish and under the weather as you did the day you began dieting. Worse, your clothes are just as tight through the midsection. Shouldn't you see some progress after a week? Aren't things supposed to change? They will if you are giving your body the fuel it needs to support its systems, rid itself of toxins, and rev up the metabolic process.

As you enter Week 2 of your cleanse you can relax, knowing that your body is working around the clock to restore its natural equilibrium. You should already be seeing significant changes in your body and in your health if you have been true to the principles of the cleanse, and particularly if you have already gone raw. You are undoubtedly feeling more energetic. The addition of increased amounts of raw food and digestive enzyme supplements to your diet means that you have started taking in the life force. At last, your body is beginning to run at full throttle, feeding on what it needs to support its systems.

If you are like most of the men and women who participate in my detox program, you are feeling healthier. Congestion, digestive problems, heartburn, aches and pains associated with chronic illness, and even the skin problems that have plagued you since adolescence may have eased or totally disappeared. Best of all, your skin may have taken on a youthful glow and clarity you haven't seen in years. This luminosity—an immediately noticeable radiance, as though a light

has been turned on inside—has attracted so many people to my classes, it has become my best advertisement. Someone notices that a friend is looking radiantly healthy and asks what she's been doing to bring about such a change. Before you know it, both friends are chugging rejuvelac and sitting in my seminar.

At the end of your first week of cleansing, you may also be rewarded with another outward manifestation of your inner transformation: a definite change in the fit of your clothes. Because of the absence of mucus-producing dairy and the addition of the fenugreek seed capsules, kamut water, rejuvelac, and other natural cleansers, you have begun to slough off the toxins that have accumulated in your abdomen, hips, and thighs. No matter what the scale says, you will feel lighter each day of this rejuvenating process, despite the fact that you are eating as much as you want, when you want.

This is the time to really check in with yourself and look for the miracles that are already occurring. In my classes in Chicago, we start Week 2 with "questions, complaints, and small and large miracles." Before students complain about a cleansing symptom, I ask them to tell me about something positive that has happened during Week 1—getting them in the habit of looking on the bright side. Whether it's in a detox class or everyday life, we need to stop leading with our complaints and start reporting all the good that is happening in our lives. We are so programmed to complain and commiserate, many of my students overlook major accomplishments until I force them to share their good news first. I ask whether they are breathing better, sleeping better, eating less, craving less sugar. Have their floaters gone away? Has their acne cleared up? The list goes on. Inevitably, every single person, even the ones most insistent upon negativity, can report some noticeable improvement in their health. These are the miracles, small and large, that prove to us that nature has the ultimate wisdom when it comes to living in true health.

MAKING THE MOST OF THE FOOD YOU EAT

In every class I teach, I have clients who are bewildered by the fact that I don't hand out specific menus. They have become so used to counting calories, carbs, or points that they have become suspicious of programs that don't restrict them. Shouldn't an expert be telling them how much they should or should not eat? I say absolutely not! You are the ultimate expert on what is best for your body, and you will instinctively know what to eat—and what not to eat—if you have faith in your body's sense of what it needs.

Like many former dieters, you may expect to be constantly hungry during this cleanse. Food cravings that you either suffer through or succumb to may have become a familiar part of your life. Nutritionists may tell you that the hunger you feel has to do with the empty, nutrient-poor calories you take in as part

of your daily diet. But that's only part of the story. Intestines that are impacted with decades of accumulated toxins cannot absorb nutrients from food. Consequently, no food you eat, whether it's three-cheese pizza or spinach salad, can possibly satisfy you. Your body craves more and more food. Before you know it, you are snacking all day long and feeling worse than ever. No wonder we're all looking for an expert to put limits on us, to keep us from eating ourselves into the next size up or the next illness.

If you are reading this book as preparation for cleansing, it may surprise you to learn that most detoxers are feeling very satisfied by the end of Week 1. Indeed, that deeply satisfied feeling is one of the most profound changes you will enjoy early in the cleanse. Oh, I can hear you now: "Satisfied? Me? Not while I'm eating rabbit food!"

If your cleanse is already under way as you read this, you will find that you are beginning to rid yourself of the intestinal plaque that has prevented you from efficiently using your nutritional fuel. You are finally getting everything you need from your food. Although you have been feasting on foods you never thought could be filling, you are becoming your own nutritional authority, drawing your intelligence from the well of wisdom you were born with and not from the latest diet books.

I now only eat when I'm hungry, and it feels amazing to have that control. I now believe I was a slave to food prior to this short course. I planned all my work meetings, family events, and entertainment around eating. I often ate for the wrong reasons. I had to put food in my body to fill the voids, not just to fuel my body. Thanks, Karyn, for releasing the chains. —J. L.

I hope that during this time you are learning the difference between "satisfied" and "full." Your stomach is not a huge receptacle to be filled to the brim three times a day. In fact, it is just a tiny sack about the size of your fist. When you eat to the point of being uncomfortable, you are stressing your digestive system and creating excess yeast and mucus in your body. On a raw diet, you are getting more nutrients from your food and can therefore be satisfied by smaller quantities.

So, have I ever had a client who, despite it all, still felt hungry throughout the cleanse? Only one. Week after week, she would appear at class, stomach grumbling. Eventually, I discovered that she was eating only salads and not including any of the healthful fats that are such a necessary part of a complete diet. When she changed her approach, she had a successful outcome.

If Week 1 of this powerful program was about making the choices that set the stage for your renewal, then Week 2 signals the advent of change. Change takes us where we need to go—sometimes abruptly. By the end of this week, you will have come to know your body as a self-renewing vehicle that delivers you to your own transformation.

LITTLE BLESSINGS: CLEANSING REACTIONS

If you have followed the Week 1 regimen, and certainly if you have begun to incorporate raw food into your diet, the mucus that lines your intestines has already started to loosen up and leave your body. You may have seen evidence of that in your stool. If so, good for you! If not, that process will certainly begin this week, along with some other common cleansing reactions. These may include bad breath, blemishes, body aches, body odor, chills, congestion or constant nasal drainage, fatigue, flulike symptoms, headaches, nausea, rashes and, most common, flatulence.

To keep a lighthearted tone, I often joke that I have led a lot of windy groups in the Windy City! As the facilitator of several hundred cleanses every year, I am well aware that flatulence and other symptoms are not anyone's idea of blessings. Cleansing symptoms, although they are to be expected and even welcomed, can be unattractive and uncomfortable. They can also be demoralizing enough to derail your cleansing effort. It is important, then, that you understand the signals your body is sending as it moves toward renewal.

Flatulence

I'm happy to report that flatulence is a common sign of candida die-off. Yeast feeds on sugars, and my cleansing program balances the sugars in your body. When you experience gassiness, you are literally blowing candida away. That's the good news.

The bad news is that it isn't easy to simultaneously celebrate this particular change in your body and maintain a social life. Cleansing symptoms are like emotions: they are best expressed, not repressed. To the extent that you can, try to adopt a "better out than in" philosophy and simply go about your normal routine. If you have a job interview scheduled or an upcoming special event, you may need to adjust your detox program to put a lid on this cleansing symptom temporarily.

Chills

Why do we associate summer eating with garden-fresh vegetables, refreshing salads, and juicy, just-picked fruits? One reason is because raw foods are known to lower body temperature.

Until I adjusted to the raw-food lifestyle, my body temperature registered around 96 or 97 degrees Fahrenheit. I felt cold all the time. If you are feeling cold during your cleanse, try adding a little ginger to your vegetable juice. If the symptom persists, sprinkle a bit of cayenne in your socks. (Just a pinch, please—too much can cause blisters.) If you are still having problems warming up to the cleansing process,

try cayenne tablets as a supplement. They help remove mucus from the system and aid in digestion, and they also work to enhance cardiac health. Another solution for the chills is to treat yourself to a long soak in a warm bath.

Skin Eruptions

Skin, your body's largest organ, releases toxins as sweat, sebum, and other natural fluids. Your skin very accurately reflects your emotional and physical condition. Needless to say, any diet change that results in the passing of larger than normal amounts of impurities will certainly affect your skin.

Our skin types are specific to each of us. Conditions that cause oily skin in one person may bring about scaliness or blemishes in another. Although cleansing will ultimately brighten and clear your complexion, you may experience some minor skin problems while accumulated toxins make their way out of your body. Keep your skin clean and moisturized, and, most of all, be patient. The oxygenated, cleansing foods you are eating are working to renew your skin from the inside out. It won't be long before your skin begins to mirror your newfound health and vitality.

Other Signs of the Time

Another side effect of detoxification is dehydration. Despite the volume of liquid you take in, you may feel dehydrated during your cleanse. You may develop bad breath, a condition that can be controlled by chewing parsley or any chlorophyll-rich food. You may develop headaches or a rash. Female detoxers can even experience some changes in their menstrual cycles. Whatever temporary inconvenience God sends to remind you that the cleanse is working, use it as a motivator, a reason to keep on keeping on.

Cleansing symptoms can be difficult to accept. People who work hard to do the right thing expect to be rewarded for their efforts. Although your temporary headaches, skin problems, or flatulence are, in a real sense, a reward, it can be hard to think of them that way. To stay focused on the positive changes you are making, share your experiences with your cleansing buddy. Together, you'll find it easier to laugh off any nuisances that come your way. After all, cleansing is a gas!

What I did on my spring cleanse: I did many things that I had never done before, like drinking wheatgrass juice, kamut water, and rejuvelac; eating dulse; and having colonics and enemas. Even though I have been a vegetarian for many years, this cleanse was a good rest from many bad foods besides meat. I had flulike symptoms and I threw up, but I got rid of a lot of toxins. My sinuses are now clearer, my back is not so stiff, I lost weight, and I don't feel like I have a rock in my stomach anymore. Most of all, I don't feel exhausted all the time. —A. P.

WEEK 2: GO RAW

Imagine that you are taking a trip and suddenly decide to change your destination. Although it took you just a moment to change your mind about where you want to go, the train cannot instantly change its route. It must be rerouted. New tracks might even have to be laid to get you to your new destination, and that will take some time and additional work.

The train journey is a metaphor for your cleansing journey. Although you have chosen to change the way you feel, it may take some time to turn your system around. You move toward your destination with every mouthful. Along the way, you may be challenged by unexpected twists in the itinerary, such as digestive upsets, headaches, or other bumps in the road. (What are naysayers if not speed bumps on the path to change?)

Days 8 through 14 are designed to kick your cleanse into high gear. Although these changes may increase your cleansing symptoms for the short term, they will also pave the way for an easier, more effective Week 3 and a smoother passage overall.

If you are still eating cooked vegan food, the time has come to go raw. So what exactly does that mean? At first when people hear about raw food, they think it means salads and carrot sticks. Nothing could be further from the truth. I could never have remained a raw foodist for over thirty years if I had to survive on bland, boring food. I need excitement, flavor, spice, and variety. When you eat raw, you choose from an abundance of vegetables, fruits, nuts, seeds, and grains. Enhanced with herbs, spices, select pure oils, and mineral-rich Himalayan and sea salts, raw foods provide a satisfying experience that is ripe with variety and exciting flavor combinations.

Nothing cleans your body, from your cellular structure to your complex physical systems, like alkalizing, fully oxygenated food. If you have not begun to sprout your own supply of easily digested, high-energy seeds and legumes, give it a try now. Sprouts are easy to grow and so delicious that many detoxers continue sprouting long after their detox is done. If you are stuck in a rut and eating nothing but tried-and-true raw food, such as salad, now is the time to try preparing raw food on your own or, if possible, stop by to learn why delicious raw meals have made my restaurant a Chicago mainstay. Well-prepared raw foods are richly flavored and deeply satisfying. They will keep you from feeling deprived. For information about sprouting and raw-food recipe books, see Resources, page 119.

In addition to removing cooked foods from your diet this week, I ask you to remove the idea that you must eat at certain times of the day. If you routinely take your meals at the same time every day, you may not be eating because you are truly hungry. Instead, you may be eating because your mind tells you it is time for break-

fast, lunch, or dinner. You may already know in your heart that this kind of thinking has contributed to your current health problems. What you might not realize, though, is that eating on schedule masks your body's hunger signals. Since one of the goals of this cleanse is to reacquaint yourself with your body and the subtle messages it sends, eating according to the clock defeats the purpose.

During this cleanse, I will not tell you when to eat or how much to eat. Consequently, it is imperative that you learn to recognize when it is time to refuel. Before you fill your plate, drink a glass of kamut water and wait a few minutes. Allow yourself the quiet time you need to listen to your body. Ask yourself if you are really hungry. Then, when you are certain about what will satisfy you, feast on as much as your body wants without guilt. For example, if you are hungry for fats, treat yourself to some sliced avocado or Almond Pâté (page 113) on raw crackers. If you crave a food you can chew, reach for a piece of fruit or some fruit leather that you've dehydrated. Over time, you will learn to give your body what it needs in precisely the amount it needs.

If you are like most of my students, you will feel more satisfied than ever on Day 8. That's because you're feeding every cell in your body in a more efficient way. Raw food is more nutrient dense and will make you feel full and satisfied, so weight loss is inevitable. The changes you make this week will turn up the heat even further, empowering you to cleanse more quickly and absorb more nutrients.

WEEK 2: WHAT'S NEW

During Week 2, build upon your progress in Week 1 by adding more raw foods, drinks, supplements, and healing therapies. The new foods and drinks are coconut oil, Energy Soup (page 112), fresh vegetable juice, and wheatgrass juice. New supplements include spirulina, a probiotic (such as Ultra Flora), and OxyKare, which is stabilized hydrogen peroxide.

During Week 2, healing therapies include daily internal cleansing. You can get colonics if you have access to and the budget for these treatments, or you can

Week 2 at a Glance

Begin a 100 percent raw vegan diet.

Continue everything you did during Week 1:

- chlorella tablets
- digestive enzymes
- fenugreek seed capsules
- gentle exercise and bodywork
- Green Meal Shake
- journaling
- kamut water
- psyllium and detox clay
- rejuvelac

Add the following:

- 2 additional tablespoons of kamut powder to your 16 ounces of kamut water
- coconut oil
- colonics or enemas followed by implants
- spirulina
- Energy Soup
- fresh vegetable juice
- OxyKare
- probiotics (Ultra Flora)
- wheatgrass juice

For a detailed summary of the Week 2 cleansing protocol, see pages 65 and 66.

give yourself enemas at home. Follow each colonic or enema with an implant of wheatgrass juice or undiluted chlorophyll liquid.

I know I am asking you to make a lot of changes this week. So be sure to read this chapter carefully before you begin Week 2 of your cleanse, then do the best you can to get everything in but do not stress about perfection. Stress will outweigh all the wonderful benefits of your detox. If you can't do everything that I recommend each day, just tell yourself that you did your best and move on. Each time I offer a detox class, I have return students. They invariably find that, although they may not have done their first cleanse perfectly, they are able to cleanse more intensely each time they detox.

Energy Soup

In my classes, I often hear this question during Week 1: "In the morning, I drink a Green Meal Shake. All day, I'm guzzling kamut water. I have to admit, I do feel full, but can't I cleanse with something that seems like food?"

During Week 2, the raw food you eat will satisfy your need to sit down at the table with the people you love most and share the bounty of the earth. In addition, you will stock your fridge with one of the most detoxifying, healing, and nourishing foods ever to grace a bowl: Dr. Ann Wigmore's Energy Soup.

The people who turned to Dr. Wigmore were often engaged in a battle for their lives. Whether her patients suffered from cancer or chronic degenerative disease, Dr. Wigmore always turned to what she called the "blessed quad" of nutrition to rebuild their worn bodies. This foursome includes the incredibly restorative Energy Soup, fresh vegetable juice, rejuvelac, and wheatgrass juice.

Energy Soup can be made in a Vitamix or another high-powered blender in just five minutes. A recipe for Energy Soup appears on page 112. I suggest that you adjust the ingredient amounts to suit your tastes and needs. Since food always turns out best when a little inspiration is included in the mix, allow your body to guide you as you choose from these wholesome Energy Soup ingredients:

DULSE: This sea vegetable is a great organic source of trace minerals in a balanced form. Dulse adds a rich, salty flavor to the soup.

REJUVELAC: This fermented drink has all the nutritional punch of sprouted wheat, friendly bacteria, and more vitamin C than orange juice.

SPROUTS: Think of them as balls of concentrated energy. Mung bean and lentil sprouts are delicious sources of fiber, iron, protein, and vitamins. They are also alive, which makes them ideal, high-enzyme additions to this wonderful soup. Select a mixture of the sprouts you like the best. Whichever you choose, you can't go wrong.

SPROUTED GREENS: Brimming with cleansing chlorophyll and filled with life-giving vitamins and minerals, sprouted greens are the foods that most directly connect us to the earth. Eating newly sprouted greens, which are fresh, nutritious, and easy to grow, is like eating the air, earth, rain, and sun that nourish them. Indeed, no food could be more naturally cleansing and energizing.

All greens are healthful. However, kale, along with buckwheat lettuce and sunflower greens (yes, I do mean the sprouted plants that will eventually grow into towering flowers), are the nutrient-packed greens that I recommend. Dr. Wigmore used to gather her own greens from whatever she found growing wild in the forest, such as lamb's quarters, purslane, and other so-called weeds. If buckwheat lettuce and sunflower greens aren't available in your area, experiment with those that are, such as dandelion greens, endive, escarole, kale, spinach, turnip greens, or watercress. All these greens will lend your soup a wonderful density of flavor and color while dramatically boosting your body's ability to cleanse.

When you're making Energy Soup, be sure not to blend the ingredients so long that they heat up. Once it's done, be sure to serve up this extraordinary meal in a manner befitting its specialness. This soup is truly the distillation of nature's essence. It deserves to be served in your best china.

WEEK 2: Begin eating Energy Soup for at least one meal each day. Because Energy Soup is a complete meal, I prefer it to salad, which is usually not made from such vital foods and can be difficult to digest. If you are feeling so full that you are having difficulty getting the soup in on a daily basis, eliminate any foods you might be eating that are not specifically on this program. Make room for what's best for you and give your body room to heal.

Wheatgrass Juice

Wheatgrass juice is a very effective detoxing agent. For most people who have tried it, wheatgrass is proof positive that human beings were meant to have the means to heal themselves, and that grass was not intended only for golf courses and picnic areas. Grown from wheat berries, wheatgrass looks similar to the grass growing in your lawn, but this simple plant has truly astounding healing properties.

Like other chlorophyll-rich foods, wheatgrass is said to cleanse the blood and the gastrointestinal tract. After drawing toxins from the blood, it builds the blood back up. It also stimulates and normalizes the thyroid gland and may be useful in correcting weight and digestive issues. Because it is so rich in chlorophyll, wheatgrass has become known as a significant anticancer agent and has even been shown to decrease the number and size of cancerous lesions in mice.

Naturally, such a powerful detoxifier elicits powerful reactions. Although some people have no negative response at all after drinking wheatgrass juice, others actually vomit after drinking it. Some gag merely at the smell. One thing is for sure: wheatgrass juice pulls out toxins—in one direction or another. For the purposes of this cleanse, that's okay. I'm sure your mother warned you about eating or drinking things that make you sick, but this is one case when it's best to make an exception. I suggest that you consider the cleansing potential in vomiting and just allow yourself to get sick.

When I first started cleansing, I could time my illness. Twenty minutes after drinking wheatgrass juice, I threw up. What could be more therapeutic? The wheatgrass was helping me clean out after twenty years of bad eating habits and drug use. If it is a challenge for you to acclimate to drinking wheatgrass juice, ask yourself what is more difficult: the daily debilitating effects of a degenerative disease or the momentary discomfort you might experience while cleansing? Then try again. I ask you to accept whatever cleansing symptoms you are blessed with. Celebrate the fact that the wheatgrass has zeroed in on something in your body that doesn't belong there.

WEEK 2: Begin your day by drinking 1 to 2 ounces of wheatgrass juice, or as much as you can tolerate, upon rising. If you are new to this amazing juice, begin drinking 1 ounce a day. If you have had it before, drink 2 ounces. I drink at least 2 ounces of wheatgrass juice every day. As soon as I've had my morning dose, I experience a wonderful sense of clarity. I'm certain you will too.

If you feel the recommended amount of wheatgrass juice is too much for you, reduce it. Just make sure you are drinking some wheatgrass juice every day. This program only lasts 28 short days. Make every one of those days count. Although you may experience some temporary discomfort, in time you will get used to the juice.

Fresh Vegetable Juice

Drinking juices made from fresh organic vegetables is the most efficient way to get nutrients into your system. When you drink the fresh vegetable juice, you are getting a compact dose of vitamins and minerals without having to put your digestive system to work. I recommend drinking juices made entirely from green vegetables. I believe that juicing with fruit or even sweet vegetables like beets can create too great a sugar rush for your system. If you simply can't stand the taste of all-green juice, it's okay to make your juice with half carrots and half greens. In a perfect world you would be drinking the vegetable juice within one hour of its being made, because the nutrients and enzymes do not remain viable much longer than that. However, this cleanse is not about perfection. It's about making

Growing and Juicing Wheatgrass

Wheatgrass is grown by sprouting organic winter wheat berries for seven to ten days and harvesting the grass when it becomes ten to fourteen inches tall. The least expensive way to obtain wheatgrass juice is by growing and juicing wheatgrass at home. Then you can cut the wheatgrass and feed it through a juicer, which separates the grass pulp from the liquid. The result is dark green juice. A bonus of growing this beautiful green grass at home is that it will oxygenate and purify any room in which it grows.

If you dedicate space in your house for trays of grass and take the time that is required to tend it, you'll have a ready source of wheatgrass to juice for mere pennies a day. There are a number of good books on the subject and equipment that will make the process easier. For more information, see Resources, page 119.

Wheatgrass juicers are sold at many natural-food stores or online through my website. The product literature or packaging should state that the machine is built specifically to juice wheatgrass. Select a high-quality juicer.

Cheap equipment won't do the job. Neither will a blender of any kind, even an expensive one. Although it may cost several hundred dollars, a good juicer is a worthwhile investment that can be used to make an amazing number of raw juices and raw foods. It will pay for itself many times over.

If you find that growing wheatgrass at home is difficult, you can purchase it from companies that ship ready-to-use wheatgrass all over the country. Many natural-food stores also sell wheatgrass for juicing. I encourage you to sample wheatgrass at a variety of stores, as growing methods and tastes can differ.

If you don't want to juice at home, you may be lucky enough to have a nearby natural-food store where you can purchase fresh wheatgrass juice daily. If not, you can buy frozen wheatgrass juice or wheatgrass powder (which is freeze-dried to preserve nutrients). Frozen or dried wheatgrass juice won't have the same properties as fresh, but it will do in a pinch.

positive changes and doing the best you can. I'm happy that you are getting vegetable juice in at all. If you are purchasing your own juicer, look for one with a double blade or twin auger. While this type of juicer is more labor intensive and time consuming to juice with, it will keep nutrients intact for at least four days.

WEEK 2: Begin drinking fresh vegetable juice, preferably made from green vegetables. Have between 8 and 32 ounces each day this week.

Coconut Oil

Coconut oil is a wonderful, healthful fat. In fact, it is a highly efficient fuel that helps your body burn fat and create instant energy. Coconut oil got an unfair rap during the early 1990s thanks to a misleading ad campaign that attacked saturated fat. But not all saturated fats are bad. The saturated fat in coconut oil, which is

very different from the saturated fat found in animal products, can raise your HDL (good) cholesterol and help to protect you against heart disease. Coconut oil boosts the immune system. Plus, it is a natural antibacterial, antifungal, and anti-inflammatory, making it highly effective in combating yeast and parasites.

WEEK 2: Begin to take 2 tablespoons of organic, unrefined coconut oil every day. Add 1 tablespoon to your Green Meal Shake. Take the other tablespoon any way you'd like. You can spread it like butter on raw crackers or raw bread, use it in a recipe, or just eat it right out of the jar by the spoonful. In chapter 4, I discuss how to use this miracle product topically as well. For more information about coconut oil, see Resources, page 119.

Spirulina

Brimming with cleansing chlorophyll, minerals, and vitamins, spirulina is a type of blue-green alga and one of the best sources of protein on the planet. Spirulina can increase endurance and mental focus; promote healthier skin, hair, and nails; and balance blood sugar levels. You are going to take powdered spirulina and make a concentrated alga water—a spirulina cocktail. Combine 16 ounces of purified water with ¼ cup spirulina powder. Pour it into a glass bottle and refrigerate. Every day you should drink 2 to 4 ounces of this spirulina cocktail. Make sure you shake it before drinking, as the powder will start to separate from the liquid. Have fun and drink it out of a shot glass—maybe one that you typically use for other types of liquids. Remember, when you first started drinking alcohol you may not have liked the way it tasted but you liked the way it made you feel. Now it's time to apply that same viewpoint to spirulina and all the other healing greens you will be taking on the program.

WEEK 2: Begin to drink 2 to 4 ounces of spirulina cocktail every day.

OxyKare

Experts have estimated that the earth's oxygen levels were 38 percent when human life was newly created. After the Industrial Revolution, those levels decreased to 22 percent. We are now living in an environment in which toxins are rampant and oxygen percentage levels in some places are in the teens. In other words, we were meant to exist optimally in an environment with 20 percent more life-giving oxygen.

In addition to the fact that we are getting less oxygen from our environment, we now get less oxygen from our food than during any time in history. In

our first days as hunter-gatherers, we subsisted entirely on fruits and vegetables. Now, a grapefruit for breakfast, an apple for a snack, and a salad for lunch might be a part of a diet that is only 50 percent raw—and the person who eats it might be considered a health nut. Since oxygen is the cornerstone of an effective cleansing program, it is important that you maximize your oxygenation during these 28 days. Adding concentrated, stabilized hydrogen peroxide to your daily regimen will help you achieve this goal.

A lot of books have been written about the role of hydrogen peroxide in the treatment of certain illnesses, including cancer. People are reporting astounding results. Food-grade hydrogen peroxide (not the kind you use for first aid) provides the kind of oxygen cells need for growth, and it is the kind that is required for the oxidation of toxins and pathogens. This preventive *and* curative one-two punch has earned it the nickname "vitamin O."

Unfortunately, most of the hydrogen peroxide products that are available in natural-food stores are unstabilized, which means you can't be certain how much active ingredient you are getting per dose. To ensure that you are getting the proper amount, I recommend that you use Karyn's Kare OxyKare Vitamin O, which I have had specially formulated. During Week 2, you will add one capful of OxyKare to 32 ounces of purified water.

If like most Americans you have been on a meat, wheat, and sugar diet for many years, you may feel quite a shock when you begin oxygenating your cells. In addition, because we hold stress, trauma, and emotional turmoil on a cellular level, you may find that some powerful emotions are unleashed once you begin to use OxyKare. Many of my clients report that they are extremely emotional during Week 2. You may become agitated, angry, short-tempered, or prone to tearfulness. Again, this is a case of "better out than in." Your mind and body are reconnecting. To stay on an even keel, journal your feelings, practice yoga, and, most important of all, never use more than the recommended amount of OxyKare.

WEEK 2: Add one capful—and *only* one capful—of OxyKare to 32 ounces of purified water. This amount of OxyKare will regenerate your cells and allow you to express yourself without risking a total meltdown. It will also work to reduce gassiness, which is a benefit that is bound to improve your mood.

Probiotics (Ultra Flora)

In today's society, many people have become crazed germaphobes. We use antibacterial soap and slather on hand sanitizers. Ironically, these products only make harmful bacteria stronger and our resistance to them weaker. But guess what? Our bodies *need* bacteria to work. The good bacteria (or microflora)

that naturally occur in our digestive tracts are essential to our digestion, nutrient absorption, and immune response. Our good-bacteria population can easily become depleted by culprits such as alcohol, antibiotics, artificial sweeteners, illness, over-the-counter medications, poor diet, stress, and travel. When our flora is depleted, digestion is compromised, potentially creating allergies and illness.

Since we spent Week 1 cleaning up our diets and beginning to flush out our digestive tracts, our intestines are primed and ready to be repopulated with friendly bacteria. In addition to eating fermented foods, such as rejuvelac and sauerkraut, supplementation is one of the best ways to do this. My Karyn's Kare Ultra Flora is a vegan probiotic supplement, free of gluten and soy, with fourteen different strains of bacteria.

WEEK 2: Begin taking three Ultra Flora capsules twice a day on an empty stomach. If you don't use my Ultra Flora, make sure you use a high-quality vegan probiotic with multiple bacteria strains.

INTERNAL CLEANSING

Imagine yourself poised on the post of a fence. I've asked you to walk across the fence, maintaining your balance some five feet above the ground. What do you do to enhance your chances of getting to the other side? If you are like most people, you use your mind to concentrate all your abilities on the task at hand. For instance, you might give yourself a mental pep talk to affirm your belief that you have the balance and concentration to make it across the fence. Or you might focus your thoughts on your goal, thus diminishing your awareness of the narrowness of the post or your distance from the ground. After your mind has been put in order, you can begin to make the physical adjustments that will bring your body into alignment with your thoughts. You might extend your arms to help you balance or change the position of your feet. Whatever your technique, you know instinctively that you cannot make it to your destination unless your mind and your body work together.

You are figuratively "on the fence" every moment of this cleanse. Whether a particular moment finds you upbeat or negative, more aware than ever of your body's potential or its limitations, you cannot achieve your goal or a healthier, more conscious life unless your mind and body are working in alignment. In my view, rebalancing is the active principle of the cleanse; it is what you do physically to strengthen the mind-body link. On Days 8 through 14, you will be rebalancing and reinforcing your cleansing efforts by adding enemas or colonic irrigation to your daily regimen.

You may be thinking, "Hey, I evacuate regularly, I don't need colon therapy!" But as we know, the human colon is very long, and waste moves through it very

slowly. If you have consumed a lifetime supply of dairy, meat, and other mucus-producing foods, you may have built up many layers of gluelike toxins on your colon walls. Although some waste can pass through your intestines daily, leading you to believe that your body is adequately digesting the food you eat, the lining of your intestines will continue to toughen and narrow. Unless you remove this toxic accumulation, your intestines will become a place where poisons are harbored deep inside your body and a source of autointoxication. You will become a source of poison to yourself.

Of course, in a world where even our own doctors don't touch us if they can possibly diagnose us with a test, it can be difficult to convince people, even those who are actively engaged in a detox, that they could benefit from going "there." If you are still skeptical, just look down. That abdominal bulge you dismiss as just another aspect of aging is a sure sign that wastes have built up in your transverse or ascending colon. Your body simply cannot use nutrients the way it should until these wastes have been removed.

The logic could not be clearer: If you eat three or four times a day, you should eliminate three or four times a day. If you do not, where have the wastes gone and what are they doing? It isn't difficult to find out. During one autopsy, a colon was discovered that was nine inches in diameter with an open passage no thicker than a pencil. Other autopsies have revealed intestines so impacted with waste that they weighed 40 pounds!

Enemas and colonic irrigation have been used for thousands of years. The Ebers Papyrus, a document dating to 1500 BC, chronicles how the ancient Egyptians used reeds to irrigate the intestines. Hippocrates used enemas to heal fevers. Ancient Romans, who made baths an obsession, considered enemas a part of good hygiene. The Essenes, who believed the body was a temple of the spirit, described an internal cleansing system using reeds and gourds to prepare their bodies to house the developing soul.

I have found internal irrigation to be almost magically curative. My clients credit this therapy for relieving their rashes and other skin disorders, and even improving their eyesight. Whatever other benefits of colon therapy you experience, it will speed the removal of toxins from your body and elevate your cleansing efforts to a new level.

After the cleanse, I lost 18 pounds of toxins and dead waste from my body. (It definitely wasn't 18 pounds of food since everything in me came out during the first two weeks.) The weight loss happened with the colonics and the fast when there was no food in my system. It was obviously all stored dead waste and toxins needing to come out. I absolutely plan on continuing cleansing and fasting twice a year or perhaps more frequently. Karyn's dedication, inspiration, and teachings have tremendously changed my life! —C. A.

Implants

As you now know, chlorophyll is a powerful detoxifying agent. What you may not know is that chlorophyll works its wonders in many ways. Used topically, wheatgrass juice can heal cuts and abrasions or be used as an effective skin cleanser. In bathwater, it increases circulation. Used in the rectum, wheatgrass juice can help pull mucus and toxins from the colon. This type of therapeutic application is known as an "implant," and it will enhance the depth of your cleanse tremendously.

If you are having colonics at a spa, ask what the procedure is for implants. Many places will charge an extra fee and require that you bring your own implant material.

If you are irrigating at home, make your own implant by blending 4 tablespoons of kamut with 4 ounces of water. Add this concentrated kamut liquid to your bucket and don't dilute with water. You can also do an implant with 4 to 6 ounces of wheatgrass juice or undiluted chlorophyll liquid. For the implant, it may be more effective to hang your bucket higher than five feet, perhaps from a hook on your shower curtain rod. Lie on your back and insert the lubricated tip into your rectum as far as it will go. Allow the liquid to flow gently into your colon. Since it is important that you hold in the liquid as long as possible to maximize the cleansing action, tip your pelvis up. Hold in the liquid for as long as you can. About twenty minutes is ideal.

Although you may expel some of the implant (along with green slimy stuff that is definitely better out than in), rest assured that this regenerating fluid is also being absorbed into your tissues, where it will work to rejuvenate your cells, rebuild immunity, and pull the poisons from your body.

WEEK 2: Follow your daily enema with an implant. If you do it before bed, the chlorophyll can work its magic while you sleep.

A FINAL WORD

For years, you've been eating the foods that your mother gave you and that are typically consumed in our society. You believed these foods were nourishing your body. Yet only now do you feel that you've come alive. During Week 2 and the remaining weeks of your cleanse, examine the following questions in your journal or your mind: What foods, specifically, do you feel have been most cleansing and energizing to you? Most importantly, how do you envision your life beyond this cleanse?

Your body is beginning to speak to you. Listen! In each burst of energy, in each clear thought, in each lost pound, your body is sending you a message. This is what it means to be well. Wrap yourself in that thought as you begin Week 3—and the rest of your life.

WEEK 2: FREQUENTLY ASKED QUESTIONS

Q: I wasn't able to do everything in Week 1 that you recommended; is it okay to move on to Week 2?

A: You are going to have to tap into your intuition on this one. Of course you can continue with the Week 1 protocol a few days longer, or even for another week, if you don't feel ready to commit to Week 2 fully yet. But if you think you are able to start incorporating the Week 2 products and therapies into your cleanse without overwhelming yourself, then go for it.

Q: I'm accustomed to drinking water all day. Although I'm getting liters of fluids and 32 ounces of water with the OxyKare, can I drink additional water?

A: Water is healing, but it won't cleanse and rebuild your cells like the green drinks. If you are still thirsty and craving water after getting in everything I recommend, then by all means, drink it.

Q: I'm drinking so many liquids that I'm having a hard time maintaining an appetite for meals. Is that healthy?

A: It's very healthy. It's a misconception that we need solid foods to sustain us. During the cleanse, what we actually live on are the gasses from the liquids we ingest. That's why everybody—from our mothers to nutrition experts—tell us to chew our foods thoroughly, until they've been liquefied. If we were supposed to swallow our food whole, we'd have teeth in our stomachs, wouldn't we?

Ingesting your food in liquid or predigested form is like taking in pure energy. You are not only providing your body with the specific type of fuel it needs, you are also providing it in a form that is easiest for the body to use. That's why so many of my clients report a sudden surge in stamina during Week 2.

It's a myth that you have to eat lots of food to provide your systems with enough necessary nutrients. In fact, craving a lot of food is often a sign that your body is starving for nutrients or that your intestines are too impacted to absorb the vitamins and minerals you eat. Normally, I take most of my nourishment as liquid. Every day I exercise, work at my businesses, and handle family matters. In the evenings, I might lead a class or speak to a group, and I usually go to bed late. Nevertheless, I get up early every morning, full of energy, and without any dark circles under my eyes. That's because I am getting everything I need from this carefully formulated diet—and so can you.

Q: Can I just mix all my liquids and powders into one "super" drink and get it over with?

A: I know it seems like I'm asking you to take in a lot at this point, and it can get overwhelming. I would like you to keep your supplements separate for a few reasons.

First, if you mixed everything together, it would taste awful. The less appealing this becomes, the less likely you are to stick with it. Second, the goal is to create new habits to replace old habits. Just like you may have reached for coffee or orange juice with breakfast, soda with lunch, iced tea as a snack, and wine with dinner, I want you to have a variety of beverages and supplements to reach for throughout the day. This will keep your interest piqued and prevent you from breaking down and reaching for a less optimal choice. That being said, you can certainly take some of your liquid and pill supplements at the same time for the sake of getting everything in.

Q: I've heard that enemas can become addictive. Is this true?

A: People who have not been having normal bowel movements or are chronically constipated often find relief during the cleanse. They can come to believe that this relief is largely due to the enemas or colonic therapy I recommend during Week 2. The truth is that this detox works to clear the colon in two ways: first, by using high-fiber, cleansing foods and supplements to sweep fecal matter and mucus from the large intestine, and second, by removing gluelike toxins from the colon walls through intestinal irrigation. Any improvement in digestion and elimination can be attributed to using both of these therapies in tandem, not to irrigation alone.

As I've said, my cleansing program is about tuning in to your body and observing the way it changes throughout these 28 days. Like most of my clients, you will find yourself drawn to raw, high-fiber foods even when this cleanse is over. They are the foods that make you feel good. They are also the foods that will work to alleviate any constipation problem you may have had.

Addiction rarely happens if you are using implants, which is why they are mandatory after every enema or colonic. If you find that you are still relying on enemas or colonics after the cleanse is through, I suggest that you carefully analyze whether it's a physical or emotional dependency. In either case, it may be a sign to seek deeper healing with a professional.

Q: Don't enemas and colonics wash away healthy bacteria?

A: Yes, they do. That's why it's important that you use implants, take your probiotics, and drink your rejuvelac. Just 16 ounces of rejuvelac every day is all it takes to restore normal bowel flora and enhance digestion. We are taking a lot out during this cleanse, but we are also putting a lot back in.

Q: I've heard about coffee enemas and implants. Do you recommend this?

A: While many people find coffee enemas and implants effective, I do not recommend them. No matter how you put it in, I don't think coffee is an optimal fuel for the body. I think it acts as a false stimulant to the colon, and who knows what negative side effects it may have. Stick with the nurturing wheatgrass juice or liquid chlorophyll, as I recommended, and you'll get great results.

TABLE 2. Week 2 protocol summary

During Week 2, you will replace your vegan diet with a raw diet and continue everything else you were doing during Week 1. In addition, begin using the supplements and therapies described in the table below.

FOOD/PRODUCT	INSTRUCTIONS	TIMING	BENEFITS
Raw diet	Eat only raw foods, which are uncooked foods, or foods that are not cooked above 118 degrees Fahrenheit (48 degrees Celsius).	Pay attention to your body's cues and eat snacks or full meals when you are truly hungry.	Raw foods are nutrient rich and the perfect choice during a cleanse. You will continue the raw vegan diet during Weeks 3 and 4.
Energy Soup	See recipe on page 112.	Enjoy this perfect meal any time of the day.	Energy Soup is an easy-to-digest, completely raw food that cleanses and rebuilds the body.
Spirulina water	Drink 2 to 4 ounces of concentrated spirulina water.	Drink every day, ideally on an empty stomach but can be taken anytime between meals.	Alkalizing, high in protein, good source of minerals and vitamins (especially B vitamins).
Wheatgrass juice	If you are unaccustomed to drinking wheatgrass juice, have 1 to 2 ounces a day. If you have had wheatgrass juice before and tolerate it well, have 3 to 4 ounces a day.	Drink these on an empty stomach, if possible, or take them anytime.	Wheatgrass juice nourishes and cleanses the body.
Fresh vegetable juice	Use a juicer to prepare fresh vegetable juice. Use all green vegetables or a mixture of ½ carrots and ½ greens. Do not use beets or fruit. Drink 8 to 24 ounces of juice per day.	Drink every day, ideally in the morning on an empty stomach.	Fresh vegetable juice is extremely easy to digest, nourishing, and alkalizing.
Coconut oil	Have 2 tablespoons of organic, unrefined coconut oil every day. Use 1 tablespoon in your Green Meal Shake and spread another tablespoon on raw crackers as a snack. Or take it by the spoonful.	Take anytime during the day.	Coconut oil is a highly efficient fuel that helps your body burn fat. It is a natural antibacterial, antifungal, and anti-inflammatory, making it highly effective in combating yeast and parasites.
Kamut water	Increase the amount of Green Kamut Powder to 4 tablespoons per 16 ounces of purified water.	Sip throughout the day.	Alkalizing, good source of vitamins and minerals, aids in healthy digestion.
OxyKare	Add 1 capful of OxyKare to 32 ounces of purified water.	Drink anytime between meals.	OxyKare is effective in treating candida and provides energy and oxygen.

(continued)

TABLE 2. Continued

FOOD/PRODUCT	INSTRUCTIONS	TIMING	BENEFITS
Probiotics (Ultra Flora)	Take 3 capsules 2 times a day.	Take on an empty stomach either in the morning or after an evening meal. Take at the onset of a headache.	Probiotics populate and promote the growth of beneficial bacteria in the small and large intestines.
Cold-milled organic flaxseed powder	Have in Flaxseed Cereal (page 110) or sprinkle on oatmeal, salad, or soup.	Use anytime during the day.	Flaxseeds are a great source of fiber and are rich in omega-3 fatty acids.
Enemas	Put 4 to 8 ounces of fenugreek water or rejuvelac into the enema bucket or bag and fill the bucket with warm water. Lie on your left side and insert the lubricated catheter tip into your rectum. Fill your colon with as much liquid as you can hold. When you can no longer hold, expel. Use all of the bucket contents. Lie on your right side and repeat the process, using another full bucket. Lie on your back and repeat the process, using another full bucket. Use no more than 3 buckets during each enema. Follow your enema with an implant (see below). *Note:* During an enema, it is helpful to rub the stomach with castor oil and place a heating pad over the oil.	Give yourself an enema or have a colonic every day. Follow either one with an implant.	Enemas remove impacted wastes and toxins.
Fenugreek water	Soak 1 to 2 cups of fenugreek seeds in 32 to 64 ounces of purified water. Let stand at room temperature for 8 to 12 hours. Strain the seeds and store the liquid in the refrigerator. Reuse the seeds once by adding more water and repeating the process.	Use for your daily enema.	Used in enemas, fenugreek water breaks down mucus and plaque.
Implants	After finishing your daily enema, add 4 to 6 ounces of undiluted kamut water, chlorophyll liquid or wheatgrass juice to the enema bucket. Lie on your back and gently insert the lubricated catheter into your rectum. (Insert the catheter as far as it will go.) Hold the liquid for 20 minutes or longer, and expel.	Use every day after your enema.	Implants work higher up in the intestinal tract than enemas. They also nourish the liver, among other organs.

Detoxing has helped me to better understand my body and what it needs to feel its best. —M.

I am not the person I was four weeks ago, and that is a good thing. I am amazed at all the changes I was able to make in such a short time. I have been able to live without bread, cheese pizza, and soda, all of my lifelong addictions, and I do not even desire to have them now. I stopped using hairspray, body lotion, and underarm deodorant. I also stopped wearing makeup, and I am amazed that people keep telling me how great I look even without it. What an accomplishment! —L. B.

I have learned so much about nutrition from Karyn. I initially took the class because I needed to take control of my life and break old habits. I will always remember the three words from Karyn that have kept me focused: keep it practical. —G.

When I began this process, I have to admit I was a bit suspicious. Only raw food? Give me a break! But less than four weeks later, the changes in the way I look and feel are so profound that I am convinced. —N. L.

During the cleanse I had to let go of what I thought I knew and open my mind to the possibility of a different lifestyle. I saw that I had burrowed myself physically and psychologically into a habit of eating and drinking for all the wrong reasons. What I learned was an entirely new way of approaching life, and I removed the psychological deadweight I had been carrying around for so long. —J. L.

I'm a business owner, a mother of two small children, a wife, and an active member of my community. I wanted to detox to prolong the quality of my life, learn an alternative way to eat, stop my migraines, and lose weight. I've achieved all my goals and so much more! —L. T.

Healing is a funny thing. Just when I thought I had achieved good health and balance, I came to realize there was yet another level of healing I could attain. Not only do I feel a whole lot healthier, I'm calmer and more present, and I have become a kinder human being. I feel more alive now than I have in years. Can you imagine—all this in just four short weeks! —C. P.

Fall has always been my favorite season. As the leaves change, I contemplate changes in my life. This fall, I was frustrated by my inability to fit into my fall wardrobe, and too proud and too frugal to purchase a new one. I was feeling sluggish and clogged. I felt a general need to cleanse my body and hoped that in the process I would also cleanse my spirit.

My boyfriend and I decided to participate in the cleanse together. It's probably good that I didn't know exactly what I was getting into before I agreed. I remember thinking, "How am I going to find enough time to do all this?" and "If she thinks I am going to give up dessert, she must be crazy."

Miracles do happen. After adopting Karyn's program, I have not craved sugar, I lost weight and increased my energy level, and I have been able to continue working out five to six times a week. Most importantly, I no longer feel polluted. —C. M.

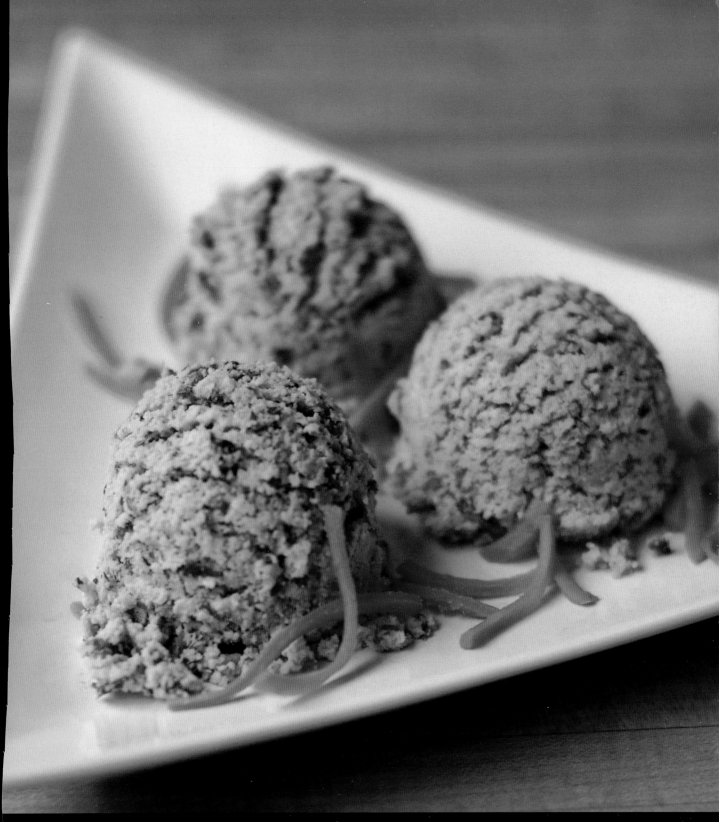

Almond Pâté, p. 113

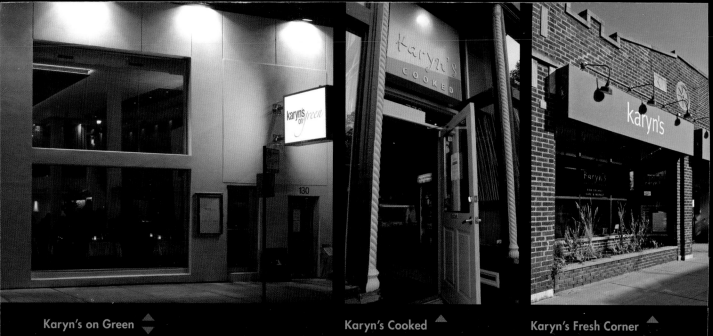

Karyn's on Green ⬍ **Karyn's Cooked** ⬆ **Karyn's Fresh Corner** ⬆

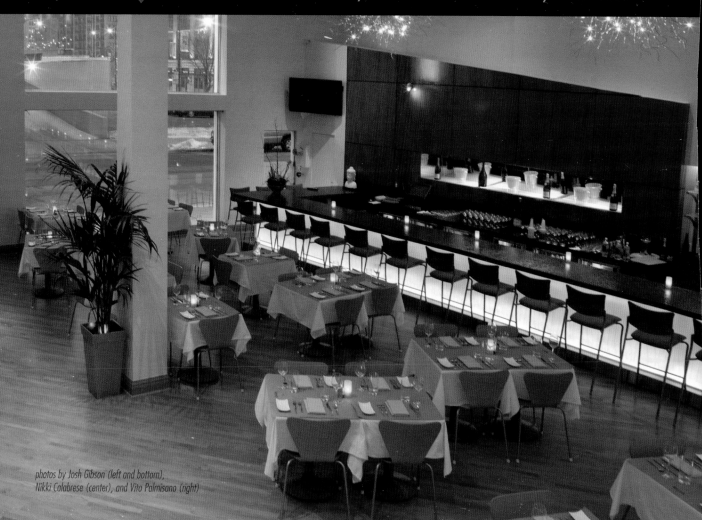

*photos by Josh Gibson (left and bottom),
Nikki Calabrese (center), and Vito Palmisano (right)*

transformation

DAYS 15 TO 21

If you have been journaling your feelings and experiences during your cleanse, the beginning of Week 3 is a wonderful time to reread what you have written. A cleanse is a growth experience, and growth can be a subtle process even if you have experienced some symptoms that made you sit back and take notice. Rereading your journal can paint a vivid picture of the person you were when you began this process. It will also remind you of the changes, both stunning and subtle, you've made in the last two weeks.

By now, the results of your hard work are really beginning to show, inside and out. You are aglow with a deep-down vitality you can't buy at any cosmetic counter. Still, the most extraordinary and exciting changes in your physical well-being might be the internal ones—the ones you can't see.

For the first time in years (perhaps since you took your first drink of cow's milk), your body is restoring itself to perfect balance. The candida you believed would always be a fact of life is diminished. Your blood sugar levels are back in check. As a result, you aren't subject to diet-busting, self-defeating food cravings anymore. The detox clay, psyllium, and enemas have removed the toxins that clogged your organs, while the oxygenated foods you are eating have bathed your every cell in pure, living nourishment. Your body feels cared for, nurtured, and alive—so much so that you may begin to feel you have reached your goal for this cleanse. In fact, you have only begun. Week 3 is the week your body has been preparing itself for. On Days 15 through 21, you will take the cleanse to its deepest level. What you will learn during these days will utterly transform the way you live in the body that houses your spirit.

PREPARE FOR TRANSFORMATION

No doubt you've already heard some discouraging words about fasting from your friends, relatives, and even casual acquaintances. Although you've never looked better and you're suddenly bursting with energy, they may tell you that what you're doing is weird and you should stop it immediately. Of course, common sense tells you that if you must make a choice between feeling well and fit and keeping company with people who don't want you to feel well and fit, then it's the people who have to go. Nevertheless, negative messages can be difficult to dismiss. You may begin to think of a hundred reasons why you cannot continue the cleanse: You are in physical discomfort. You are having emotional outbursts that make those around you feel uncomfortable. Or maybe your spouse, children, or lifestyle won't "allow" you to complete the good work that you have started.

Whether it's emotional, psychological, or physical, self-improvement is hard, dirty work. And the work gets harder before it gets easier. You don't need much imagination to come up with lots of reasons to quit working. I've stopped a few cleanses for lousy reasons myself. But more times than I've hit the wall of my own negativity, I've crashed right through. Now I'm here to tell you that these "reasons" are not reasons at all. They're excuses. You've already invested two full weeks in your own health and longevity. All you need to do now is hang on a little longer to reach new heights of cleansing. As for any physical discomfort you may be experiencing, congratulations. Strong cleansing reactions mean that you are doing the work. With determination and luck, you may experience even stronger symptoms in the next few days. Meanwhile, let's examine some of the common experiences that detoxers report during Week 3 of the cleanse.

Rectal Soreness

Are you sitting down? If you're not, your enema and implant technique might be taking its toll! Before beginning your next treatment, make certain that you are lubricating the catheter tip very well before insertion. Then, between enemas, treat yourself to a series of warm baths or sitz baths.

The skin and tissue around the anus is very sensitive. They are also prone to cleansing symptoms. When you are using implants or enemas, make sure that you are taking the time to nurture your body. Don't rush; proceed slowly, at your body's own pace. Allow yourself plenty of time to relax, to "go with the flow" of the healing fluids you are introducing. These treatments are deeply curative therapies that have been used successfully for thousands of years. Any associated discomfort can usually be alleviated with a small adjustment in position or technique.

When I first started cleansing, I experienced rectal soreness and severe pain from hemorrhoids. I saw it as part of my healing crisis and powered through it. That may be the right path for you as well. However, if you are experiencing pain or any extreme discomfort, do what feels right to you, even if that means stopping the enemas or colonics.

Dry Skin

Now that you have reduced the toxic buildup in your colon, your food is moving through your digestive system more quickly. As a result, your skin may feel a bit drier than usual. If it does, add some avocado, seeds, or nuts to your diet to replace some of the fats that are being swept away by the psyllium and detox clay. You might also lubricate from the inside out by adding another tablespoon of flaxseed oil or coconut oil to your Green Meal Shake.

Your skin is your largest excretory organ. That means that during this powerful cleanse, huge amounts of toxins are being released through your pores. This may be drying to your skin. Since the detoxing process reaches its height during Week 3, we will begin some topical treatments to help the skin remove any accumulated poisons quickly and effectively (see page 98).

During the cleanse, I "paid the piper" in feelings of depression, fatigue, cramps, and mood swings. However, now I feel that I am finally seeing the end of the tunnel—and I like the view! Not only have I witnessed physical changes in my body, but I am also becoming more independent in my thinking and a little more focused on finding my purpose in life. This program has been just as much a spiritual journey as a physical one. —**B. B.**

Weight Gain

I know it's hard to believe, but some people actually gain weight during the first few weeks on this program. This is particularly true of detoxers who suffer from very pronounced candida growth. You may experience weight gain if you came into the program with a yeast imbalance or if you have been eating a lot of raw desserts or sugary foods, such as fruit or starchy vegetables. Rest assured that weight gain is a temporary condition. The Week 3 regimen will certainly take care of this problem.

The beauty of this cleanse is that it is not a diet—it is a transformation. In contrast, diets are temporary regimens, programs that we start on Monday and stop when we can squeeze into our skinny pants. When we diet, we don't really change our eating habits. Since most diets are based on foods that we were never intended to eat, such as meat, dairy, and artificial sweeteners, they certainly cannot make any biochemical changes in our bodies.

Because it is based on the pure, oxygenated nourishment nature intended for us, Nature's Healing System works on a cellular level to restore the body to

its own standard of perfection. This cleanse will help you where you need it the most. For example, detoxers who need to throw off fat might lose 20 pounds in two weeks. Those who have yeast to work on might rid themselves of candida but lose little weight.

Whatever challenges you face, I guarantee that Week 3 will hasten your cleansing and put your body into complete balance. It will also heighten your awareness of how your body is healing itself through this purifying process. Your body knows exactly what it needs for optimal performance. Although those extra pounds might be a weighty emotional issue for you now, your body can only correct its imbalances by working through the cleansing process. Trust your body's wisdom. This cleanse may set the stage for permanent weight loss later on.

Chills, Cramping, Fatigue, and Other Cleansing Symptoms

Remember the *Saturday Night Live* character, Roseanne Roseannadanna? She could reel off a list of physical complaints longer than *The Merck Manual*. She might report, in her characteristic singsong, that she was suffering from aches, bloating, boils, chills, cold sores, cramps, flatulence, goose bumps, migraines, night sweats, rashes, and even a little ball of sweat clinging to the end of her nose. So what do Roseanne's twinges, throbbings, and uncontrollable emissions have to do with you? During Week 3, you are probably still carrying over some healing symptoms from last week. And you are probably ready to unleash your own list of complaints, Roseanne Roseannadanna–style.

I will repeat that cleansing reactions aren't run-of-the-mill inconveniences. They are your body's way of telling you that it is bringing itself back into balance. While it is tempting to pop a pill that will temporarily mask your body's messages, haven't you been self-medicating with the wrong foods, unnecessary drugs, and harmful chemicals long enough? Didn't the very foods, such as ice cream, processed foods, and sugary snacks, that you hoped would make you feel better bring you to your current condition in the first place?

Most of the people who don't complete this program, and they are few, don't make it because they don't acknowledge their healing crises the right way. One way to make things easier is to divorce yourself from the quest for instant relief. Whether you're talking about pregnancy, growth, or healing, every biological process happens at its own rate. Your cramps or fatigue aren't just cleansing symptoms; they're growing pains. And growing pains are nothing more than God's little reminders that He is working a miracle in your body. When aches or pains or odors happen, be in your body. I mean *really* sink into it. Feel what it's like to live in your skin, right here, right now. Visualize the work your body is doing to rid your system of toxins. Be grateful for these signs that your organs

are doing their job and welcome those that are still to come. They are the side effects of a life worth living.

Cleansing is a journey with many twists and turns. As you begin the last half of this adventure, I want to remind you not to let yourself be deterred by any emotional symptoms of detoxification that you experience. We swallow a great deal of what ails us when we engage in emotional eating. Divesting ourselves of our toxic emotions and the toxic foods with which we tried to soothe them is a challenge to both mind and body. During some of my cleanses, I've fought and argued with everyone around me. I've cried my way through others, either out of anger or profound grief.

During these 28 days, when you find yourself struggling to maintain your emotional composure, do yourself a favor: don't. Have a heart-to-heart talk with your cleanse buddy, scream, punch a pillow, write in your cleansing journal, or pour out your feelings in a letter (which, I caution you, you may not want to send). Allow yourself to connect with the emotions that are surfacing during your cleanse. Emotional eating is about masking. If you could not feel the power of your emotions when they were on their way in, it is important that you experience them as they are on their way out. If you can become conscious of the feelings, such as anger, envy, and resentment, that you tend to swallow, you will be less apt to carry this self-defeating habit into the future.

WEEK 3: WHAT'S NEW

If we compare the cleanse to the Olympics, Weeks 1 and 2 were about training and preparation. Week 3 is the main event. This is also the week when miracles happen.

If you've attended my cleansing seminar or read any of the testimonials that appear in this book, you know that real miracles—relief from lifelong chronic conditions, the disappearance of symptoms, and even complete cures—are common occurrences for detoxers. I could fill a book with my clients' inspiring stories. For example, Joyce, who lived across the street from my restaurant, couldn't make it up my stairs before her cleanse. Donna suffered from benign tumors that totally dissolved. John, who has HIV, saw his T cell count increase from 250 to 850 in just twenty-one days. These miracles and the dozens of others chronicled in this book are a testament to the body's amazing ability to renew itself when given half a chance. This week, you will give your body that chance.

What will you remove from your diet on Days 15 to 21? For four days out of the seven, nothing. On these days you will continue the Week 2 protocol. The other three days you will devote to the ultimate healing tradition: fasting.

The Fast

Fasting is an integral part of all the world's major religions. For thousands of years, mystics of all spiritual traditions have relied on fasting to cleanse their bodies and souls, free their focus from the body's mundane needs, and prepare themselves for the grace of illumination. Mahatma Gandhi credited fasting as a powerful means to attaining spiritual enlightenment and affecting positive change. It is important to recall that the benefits of going without food aren't just spiritual; they are also intellectual and corporal.

History shows that both Plato and Socrates fasted regularly to build mental and physical efficiency. The medical literature of ancient China, Egypt, Greece, and Rome all agree on the curative benefits of fasting. Supporters of fasting today report that a controlled fast of a suitable duration is effective in the treatment of a great number of conditions, including allergies, arthritis, asthma, heart problems, intestinal irregularities, insomnia, migraine headaches, rashes, sinus disorders, skin eruptions, stomach ulcers, thyroid abnormalities, tumors, and vision problems such as cataracts and glaucoma. In addition, during the last century scientists have concretely established the link between eating less and living longer. Researchers who follow this thread today seem destined to retrace the footsteps of the knowledgeable medical pioneers of long ago.

To clarify, fasting is not starving. It is the process of doing without food (but not fluids!) long enough to allow the body to purge itself of accumulated toxins. After an effective, cleansing fast, metabolic order is reestablished. People emerge feeling energized, intellectually focused, and vibrantly alive. Fasting is a truly transformative and life-affirming experience that most people are eager to repeat. Remember, we have not gone from eating everything to fasting overnight. We have been preparing our bodies for two weeks for this part of the cleanse. We have been eating less, balancing our blood sugar, ridding our bodies of toxins, and much more. It is very important that you never just stop eating and fast without preparation.

No doubt you are aware that there are many different types of fasts. There are, for example, juice fasts, water fasts, and even fasts that are limited to a single type of food, such as brown rice or fruit. Since the word "fast" is derived from the Old English word *faestan*, which means "go without food," single-food regimens are not technically fasts at all. A true cleansing fast works in two ways: first, it encourages the deepest possible detoxification through the purging of toxins and mucus from the body, and second, it allows the body a break from the energy-consuming business of digestion, thus encouraging it to heal.

For our purposes, the fast will be a liquid-based diet that consists mainly of highly oxygenated green drinks, nourishing vegetable juices, powerfully revitalizing wheatgrass juice, and rejuvelac. If you have never fasted before, I suggest

Is Fasting Normal?

Cindy, a student in one my seminars, wasn't so sure. Although she had come through the first two weeks of the cleanse with flying colors, when she was faced with the prospect of the fast, she said, "Karyn, I've followed this program to the letter for two weeks, and I've never felt better. Still, I just can't get over the idea that going without food even for a few days just isn't normal."

Her comment prompted a few chuckles from the class, but Cindy had brought up an important issue. Judging from the waist measurement of most businessmen's pants, fasting is *not* normal in the United States. It certainly is not in Chicago, my hometown, which is known as a great place to chow down. What is normal? For most Americans, normal is a cardboard boat filled to the point of capsizing with two thousand calories of fries and cheese—and that's a snack! It's also normal for us to experience food as reward, food as love, food as obsession, food as anything but what it is really supposed to be: nourishment. In that light, going without food altogether is certainly not what we call "normal." Or is it?

To understand normal behaviors, scientists often look to animals, who have remained in touch with their instincts. When they are sick, animals go without food. Passing up the feed conserves strength and gives vital systems a much-needed break. Fasting allows whatever energy the sick animal has to be used for healing. So while humans equivocate about whether the old adage goes starve a fever, feed a cold, or vice versa, animals do what comes naturally.

Think of your body as a piece of machinery. If you have been eating three squares daily, you have been running your machine twenty-four hours a day for as many decades as you have been alive, just to move that food through your system. This fast is your chance to shut down your machine, see where restoration is necessary, and begin rebuilding.

After years of cleansing, I no longer experience healing crises or weight loss while fasting. My weight, energy level, and emotions remain in balance. Since the fast will be a deeply cleansing period for you, you may experience one or more detoxing symptoms, including light-headedness, flulike symptoms, emotional upset, or any of the mild aches and pains you may have experienced earlier on. Make no mistake—you have entered the ultimate cleansing zone. Having carefully prepared your body during the last two weeks, you are now reaching into your innermost recesses. The toxins that are being released into your system have been embedded there for years. Instead of malingering or focusing on any symptoms you may be experiencing, think about how the poisons were able to take up residence in your system in the first place. What was God's intention for you: to be a chemical dumping ground or the self-healing miracle He created? Every day of this fast, you are moving toward God's intention.

that you maintain this regimen no longer than three days. That being said, I have had first-time detoxers who have fasted much longer than three days. If you feel you are really listening to your body and can keep fasting, by all means do so. Just don't push yourself too far. Know when it's time to gently break your fast. Of course, if you are an experienced detoxer who has completed my program before, you can trust your intuition about how long to fast. You have learned enough about your body to know what it feels like when it is working at peak efficiency.

Oil of Oregano

When you use this deeply healing herbal tincture during your fast, it will give you results beyond your wildest imagination. Because oil of oregano is extremely concentrated and potent, the smell and taste may turn you off at first. However, once you get beyond first impressions, you will be blown away by the healing power of this supplement. During times of high stress, oil of oregano is the first thing I grab for its immediate calming effect. Its natural antibiotic properties fight colds, funguses, parasites, viruses, and yeasts. Oil of oregano is also a natural anti-inflammatory and very healing for digestive disorders. If this supplement is too much for you at first, you can start with one or two drops a few times a day and build your tolerance gradually; but remember, we are in boot camp right now. The more you are able to do, the more powerful your results will be.

WEEK 3: Take one dropperful once or twice each day that you fast.

Systemic Enzymes

This is one of the supplements that has truly changed my life. As we learned earlier in the book, enzymes are responsible for every metabolic purpose in your body. Digestive enzymes work specifically in the stomach and intestines to help the body digest food, absorb nutrients, and relieve gastrointestinal disorders. Systemic enzymes strengthen the body as a whole by passing through the digestive system and targeting tissues and organs. They are always taken on an empty stomach so that they are not tied up in the digestive process, negating their true power.

Systemic enzymes stimulate the immune system and can relieve common ailments, like sinus congestion, headaches, and arthritis. They can also improve circulation, reduce inflammation, and break up cholesterol and fibrin in the blood vessels. You will notice increased flexibility and reduced soreness while taking these enzymes. Some of the doctors who have taken my class prescribe large doses of systemic enzymes for their patients who have suffered from athletic injuries and they see fabulous results. In my sixties, I still take professional-level ballet classes with girls in their teens. Thanks to systemic

I must admit, I was skeptical about the idea of a hypoglycemic fasting. The two just don't go together. Everyone said it couldn't be done. They were wrong! I did a successful three-day fast and I am now working on Day 21 of being free of dairy, sugar, meat, and wheat. I have a burst of energy, I feel lighter, and I have had no blood sugar reaction. This is a lifestyle change for me. I'm not going back. —S. J.

enzymes, I find that my toes don't callous and my body bounces back faster than most of those "spring chickens"!

I'm making this enzyme an optional choice for the cleanse. I realize that you have probably already devoted a lot of money to this process and the systemic enzymes may not be in your budget. If you can afford it, though, I highly recommended them. They are something I can't live without, and I know the same is true for many of my clients. If you don't take the systemic enzymes during this cleanse, you can begin taking them whenever you are ready.

WEEK 3: Take three capsules twice a day during the fast. Can be continued after the fast as well.

Week 3 at a Glance

Begin the following:
- the fast (three or more days)
- oil of oregano
- systemic enzymes (optional)

Stop the following (while fasting):
- solid food
- Energy Soup
- fenugreek seed capsules
- Green Meal Shake
- psyllium and detox clay

Continue the following:
- 100 percent raw diet when not fasting
- colonics or enemas and implants
- spirulina water
- fresh vegetable juice
- kamut water
- water with OxyKare
- rejuvelac
- wheatgrass juice

The following are optional:
- coconut water
- digestive enzymes
- energy therapy
- oxygen bathing
- probiotics (Ultra Flora)

Try the following:
- bathe in sea salt
- brush your skin
- detox your home
- detox your tongue
- eliminate antiperspirant or deodorant
- moisturize with olive or coconut oils
- practice healing breath work
- use natural soaps

For a detailed summary of the Week 3 cleansing protocol, see page 88.

WEEK 3: WHAT STOPS

During the fast, you will stop eating all "chew food," by which I mean solid foods that you must grind with your teeth to get down. You will also stop eating Energy Soup, taking fenugreek seed capsules, and drinking the Green Meal Shake and your psyllium-detox clay cocktail.

WEEK 3: WHAT CONTINUES

During your fast, it is essential that you continue colonics or enemas and implants. In addition, continue the juices and supplements during your fast. They will boost your body's ability to heal without taxing your digestive system.

Colonics, Enemas, and Implants

It's the question I knew had crossed the minds of everyone in the seminar room. But it took Mike, an outspoken salesman, to ask: "I know you say 'better out than in,' but now that there's nothing going in, what could possibly come out? Do I still have to do the enemas and implants during the fast?"

I'd be the first to agree with Mike if there really wasn't anything to come out during the fast. However, your fast is a time of maximum cleansing. More toxins than ever are being flushed from your body. Think about it. When political prisoners go on a fast, what do they die of? Not starvation. They die of toxemia caused by the rush of toxins into their systems. Therefore, to keep the poisons moving out of your body, it is more important than ever that you have an enema or colonic every day and follow it with an implant.

To put it another way, if you aren't willing to have the enemas or colonics, it's best that you don't fast. Coaxing toxins into your system during a fast and then not flushing them away can be dangerous, especially when your body is at its most vulnerable. If you've come this far, why not go all the way? Colonic therapy might cause you a little discomfort now, but it's nothing compared to the health problems you could experience for years to come if you don't do it.

Fresh Vegetable Juice

Continue drinking green juice; that is, fresh vegetable juice made from green vegetables or from half green vegetables and half carrots. During a fast, your heart works hard to rid your body of toxins. You may even notice your heart pounding from time to time. By flushing your system with fresh, nutrient-rich vegetable juice, you enhance the body's ability to maintain strength and energy while moving out the toxins. It's important that you don't fast on any other sweet vegetables (like

beets) and absolutely have no fruit juices or sweeteners. While cleanses that recommended fasting with maple syrup or honey have become very popular, I have to strongly caution against that practice. Taking in large amounts of sugar during a fast can overwhelm the spleen and imbalance blood sugar. In my experience, this leads to strong sugar cravings and unwanted weight gain after the fast is over.

Green Kamut Powder

Continue drinking your kamut water. If you haven't already done so, it's time to increase the amount of Green Kamut Powder. Double the amount by mixing 4 tablespoons of green kamut powder in 16 to 32 ounces of purified water.

OxyKare

Continue but do not increase the amount of OxyKare you use this week. One capful in 32 ounces of purified water will do the trick. More is not always better.

Rejuvelac

Continue to drink as much rejuvelac as you'd like throughout the day. Nothing will help you maintain your energy during a fast like rejuvelac.

Wheatgrass Juice and Spirulina

For optimal results, continue to take 2 to 4 ounces of *both* spirulina water and wheatgrass juice every day during your fast. As I said, this cleanse is like the Olympics. Shoot for the moon, but do what you can.

This was truly an interesting detox for me. Everything felt so natural. Then it dawned on me that this way of living is becoming more and more a part of my lifestyle. I am truly proud of my four-day fast. Next time, I am going for five days!

—T. T.

Digestive Enzymes and Probiotics

Many people find it difficult to swallow pills when they are fasting. However, if you are able to do so, continue taking your digestive enzymes and probiotics (Ultra Flora). Taking digestive enzymes with your green juice can enhance nutrient absorption. After an enema or colonic, the Ultra Flora will help to quickly replenish good bacteria in your system.

TIPS FOR A SUCCESSFUL FAST

Although it is part of the larger process of cleansing, you will find that the fast will seem to take on a life and character of its own. Because fasting is experienced on both the physical and spiritual planes, it may lead you to inward

Benefits of Fasting

Fasting sometimes gets a bad rap—mostly from people who've never experienced it. The truth is, there is no experience more centering, more physically and spiritually cleansing, than a few days respite from food. Ask anyone who has given himself over to the discipline of fasting and he will tell you that going without food can be the best medicine. Even a brief fast allows the body and mind to clear, bringing the following benefits:

- deeper sleep
- enhanced immunity
- greater spiritual awareness
- improved complexion
- inspiration
- longevity
- more energy
- reduced allergies
- relaxation
- weight loss

pursuits, such as meditation, automatic writing (a practice of writing in a journal any thoughts that come into your mind, even if what you write is a complete ramble), or any contemplative practice. You will also experience myriad physical passages, some of which can be challenging.

Like many of the men and women who participate in my detox program, you might find yourself breezing through your first day without chew food. People tend to psyche themselves up for a fast. Expecting the worst, they lay in supplies to help them get through the experience. They line up their fluids like soldiers in the refrigerator, they surround themselves with uplifting reading material, and they may schedule a massage or some other body-work to reward themselves for their persistence. Then comes Day 2. Twenty-four hours in, the newness of the fasting experience has worn off, along with some of that newbie enthusiasm. You may feel tired, irritable, distinctly unspiritual, or extremely hungry. Needless to say, at times like this, even the toughest totally vegan, dehydrated-not-baked cookie can crumble—unless he or she has a plan.

Obviously, for these very short three days, it is best that you stick with the fast. The ongoing effects of this intensely cleansing time will reward you for months to come. If, however, you feel so famished that you fear you will abandon the fast entirely, you have some options:

- **Drink some rejuvelac.** The protein in this wondrous drink might be just the thing to quiet your hunger pangs.

- **Drink coconut water.** This is especially helpful if you crave something sweet. If possible, drink fresh and unpasteurized water straight from a coconut. However, the packaged variety will do the trick as well.

- **Indulge in a cup of Energy Soup.** It's the right choice if the rejuvelac and coconut water are not enough, and you're still teetering on the edge. But make no mistake. Energy Soup is a whole food. It may look like a liquid, but it still has fiber. Consuming it will put your digestive system to work. If you treat yourself to a helping, you are technically no longer fasting. Still, if the soup helps you get back on track and gives you the willpower to make it through another day of the fast, this small lapse is well worth it. Besides, breaking the fast with Energy Soup is distinctly preferable to chowing down on pepperoni pizza or anything else that will derail your cleanse.

PROTECT AND PAMPER YOURSELF

The body works hard during a fast. Although you may feel more alive and energetic than ever, your body may be more vulnerable to illness than at any other time. Consequently, the fasting period is not a time for strenuous exercise or hard work. It is a time to nurture and honor the magical vessel that harbors your spirit.

During these three days, allow your body the time it needs to adjust to the fast and rebalance. Treat yourself to long walks, use a mini trampoline to encourage lymphatic drainage, and try to find time in your day to reinforce the crucial relationship between your body and your mind. Devote an hour to yoga (but not ashtanga, Bikram, or any other physically demanding type). Meditate on the miracle that is occurring within you. Despite the abuses it has endured, your body is working very hard to cleanse itself and provide you with longevity and vigor.

The fasting period can be an incredibly empowering time. Feel yourself taking back control over your life. With every hour that passes, your focus, fortitude, and potential increase. You regain your power. You can further enhance this position of power and this positive viewpoint by fasting from all media during this time. Avoid the television news, newspapers, and online news sites. What are they but daily delivery systems for bad news? Cleanse them from your consciousness. Better yet, replace them with some deliciously enlightening reading. I suggest *The Joy Book* by Prem Raja Baba. This powerful book ushered me into new levels of understanding about my life. Or try *The Golden Present* by Swami Satchidananda for daily inspiration.

You will find the fast to be a deeply healing time. How could it be otherwise? You are giving your body precisely what it needs to be at its best. Nothing could be more nurturing. In return, your body is giving you a profoundly reassuring sense of physical and spiritual well-being. Don't be surprised if your sleep patterns are thrown off during the fast. You may sleep more than ever before, or you may require very little sleep. You may be wide awake at three in the morning and feel fatigued at three in the afternoon. Don't worry about the changes—they are only temporary. Listen to your body as much as possible and give it what it needs. It may be best to fast over the weekend when you don't have as many obligations to fulfill.

When you fast, you are very vulnerable to chemicals and toxicity. Just as you have eliminated toxicity from your diet and focused on the oxygen-rich foods that feed your cells, you also want to pay close attention to the products that you are using on your skin. Remember that everything you put on your skin is absorbed directly into your blood stream and affects you the same way as food. To make the most of this special time, consider some of the following changes to eliminate topical toxins.

Eliminate Antiperspirant or Deodorant

The lymph nodes, many of which are located in your armpits, collect toxins and need a rest from the constant onslaught of chemicals they absorb. Your sweat flushes wastes from your body. If you stop the flow of sweat with antiperspirants, you block your body's natural ability to cool and clean itself. Just this once, let it all hang loose! You'll be surprised at how clean your natural, untreated skin can smell. If you are still insecure, pick up a natural deodorant at your local natural-food store. Alternatives to toxic deodorant solutions work like crazy without blocking pores or compromising health. Meanwhile, consider this: after several detoxes, when you are really clean, your healthy perspiration won't smell like decomposing meat or old chemicals anymore. Like me, you'll be antiperspirant and deodorant free. And, trust me, I still have close friends.

Opt for Gentle Cleansing

Most soaps are very drying and full of additives and chemicals. Particularly during the fast, it is important that you clean and care for your skin by using a natural soap. It may cost a little more than the mass-produced product you're currently using, but it will leave your skin clean, soft, and chemical free.

Moisturize Naturally

Fasting offers incredible potential for internal hygiene. It makes no sense, then, to coat your skin with lotions or moisturizers that contain chemicals or perfumes. You can help your skin do its job by lubricating it with a natural product. To keep my skin supple every day, I depend on olive oil or coconut oil. I keep them in pump dispensers in my bathroom so they're always within reach. Although I've been through menopause (so my skin should be dried up, right?), my skin has the texture and feel of a baby's.

You can experiment with sesame oil as well. A mainstay of the ancient ayurvedic tradition, a massage with sesame oil is believed to relieve stress, stimulate and cleanse the skin, and bring energy and alertness to the entire body. To massage in accordance with ayurvedic tradition, move the oil in long strokes along your bones and in a circular pattern at your joints.

Brush Your Skin

Skin brushing is a technique dating back thousands of years. It is known to aid the skin in its effort to excrete accumulated poisons and promote exfoliation.

When you are in the bathroom for your enema or before your shower, take a soft brush and start stroking your dry skin. Begin with your head and neck,

and then move to your extremities, always working toward your heart. Not only will the stimulation awaken your every nerve ending, it will also sensitize and stimulate your skin, prompting even deeper levels of detoxification.

Bathe in Sea Salt

If you feel done in by the rigors of the day, or if you're just being especially kind to yourself during this time, try a therapeutic bath. Add 2 or 3 pounds of sea salt to a tub of warm water and soak your cares away. The salts will pull the toxins from your system and remineralize your bones. This is an especially rewarding option if you're experiencing soreness or achy muscles as a cleansing effect.

Detox Your Tongue

In the ayurvedic tradition, the tongue is examined in order to diagnose illness. For five thousand years, ayurvedic doctors have recognized the presence of a white coating on the tongue as an indication of toxicity in the system due to improperly digested food. Whether you give credence to ancient Indian theory or not, you can be sure that poisons and toxins will make their way out of your system through your mouth and tongue during this intensely cleansing week. To keep this great benefit from leaving a bad taste in your mouth, scrape your tongue regularly to remove any bacteria that have accumulated there.

Although you can use any dull blade, such as a butter knife or the edge of a teaspoon, I recommend that you invest in a tongue scraper. (They are designed with a little hook on the end that really gets the job done.) Gently scrape your tongue from back to front a dozen or so times until the entire surface is clean. This simple technique will keep your breath fresh and prevent you from swallowing the toxins you have succeeded in removing.

Since commercially produced toothpaste is filled with artificial flavorings and added chemicals, it would be wise to eliminate it from your daily regimen. Do you really want to use a product that warns "keep out of reach of children" right on the package? If you want to switch to a more natural product, I recommend my Karyn's Kare Miracle Toothpaste. Brush well at least twice a day to keep toxins from announcing their presence.

Detox Your Home

Commercial household cleaning supplies are full of so many toxic chemicals, it is widely believed they are causing asthma and allergies in children. Lucky for us, a great variety of chemical-free and highly effective household cleaning supplies are available. In fact, simple white vinegar and baking soda are excellent and nontoxic household cleaners.

During this week, cleaning products will surely come in handy because, either during the fast or after, you will experience a burst of energy that you haven't felt since childhood. You may be inspired to clean your cupboards, sort your closets, or tackle some other major project. (In fact, I wrote the first draft of this book when I was on a thirty-day fast.) Many of my clients report that immediately following the fast they are driven to re-create in their external lives the order that they feel within. Take advantage of this feeling. Clean house. Get rid of a few pairs of those slimming black pants that are taking up room in your closet. They probably don't fit you anymore, anyway.

ENHANCE YOUR FAST WITH ALTERNATIVE THERAPIES

Perhaps more than any other practice, fasting draws us into our very essence, where reality is not about meetings or schedules or responsibilities but about the natural harmony between the nurtured body and the conscious mind. Needless to say, you may want to reach beyond the ordinary to care for yourself during this special time. Following are a couple of therapies that I recommend.

Oxygen Bathing

As we have already discussed, oxygen levels in our atmosphere have dropped from 40 percent during the time of the dinosaurs to as low as 11 percent in highly industrial areas today. Eating foods that are low in oxygen and exposing ourselves to pollutants have made our bodies fertile breeding grounds for a host of opportunistic diseases, including arthritis, cancer, chronic fatigue syndrome, multiple sclerosis, and many more.

A great way to reoxygenate the body is hydrotherapy with an oxygen bath or aerobic spa. These baths employ temperature-controlled oxygenated water to soothe and warm the body, removing the toxins that are released by perspiration more effectively than plain water or steam. This action can improve digestion, stimulate the immune system, support heart health, and increase overall relaxation. The oxygen bath works wonders. Natural-health centers across the country are beginning to discover the lasting benefits of this profoundly rejuvenating therapy.

Infrared Sauna

Bask in the warmth of an intensely healing infrared sauna. Unlike traditional dry saunas, these saunas use infrared technology to push toxicity from the body. Mimicking the rays of the sun, infrared technology can penetrate deep into your skin and actually get to work on your body's systems. Infrared has been shown to detox heavy metals and trans fats from the organs. Thirty minutes a day in an infrared sauna is like get-

ting in a three-mile run or intense gym workout without the effort! In a traditional sauna you will sweat out about 5 percent toxins and 95 percent water, whereas in an infrared sauna, you will sweat about 15 percent toxins and 85 percent water. If you don't have access to an infrared sauna, a traditional sauna is a suitable alternative.

Energy Therapy

Every living thing vibrates as energy. Frequency, the specific level of vibration emitted by a source, is the language of energy. In order for the body to be healthy, energy must flow freely throughout it. The Rife machine, also known as a Bio-Ray, is a vibrational energy therapy that applies frequency information, including color, electricity, light, sound, and subtle and magnetic energy, directly to the body to break up blockages, energize the lymphatic and circulatory systems, and create perfect alignment between the body and mind.

This marvelous machine eradicates blockages to restore vitality to the energetic channels. The body can then heal itself of a host of problems, including, it is believed, cancer. For more information about the benefits of this therapy, read *The Cancer Cure that Worked* by Barry Lynes. Although I make no specific claims, I can tell you that in general, if your health is compromised, vibrational energy therapy will help. If you are well, it will boost your overall health. This form of therapy may not be easy to find. However, some alternative-healing centers, including mine, have them. If you can't find a BioRay near you, try qigong or another form of energy work.

BREAK YOUR FAST GENTLY AND CAREFULLY

As we have discussed, fasting is an active principle in most of the world's religions. For thousands of years, fasting has also been used as a therapeutic discipline, a preventive measure to put the body back into its natural balance, and a curative that has been successfully applied to a host of diseases. Considering the long history of this respected practice, you will find there are nearly as many suggested ways of breaking a fast as there are reasons to fast.

Follow my instructions on breaking your fast to the letter. I will ask nothing of you that is more important during this entire program. At this point, your body is at its most vulnerable. In this moment lies the greatest potential for healing or serious discomfort.

The best foods to eat after you've finished a fast are the same easy-to-digest, oxygen-rich foods you were eating in preparation for it. That means breaking your fast with a delicious, revitalizing bowl of satisfying Energy Soup. Later in the day, when hunger hits, you can have more Energy Soup or, if you're ready to chew, move on to a sprout salad. Sprouts are an easily digested, living food. Feasting on

a blend of alfalfa, clover, or sunflower sprouts will gently reawaken your digestive system without stressing it. You will ease back into eating by feeding your body precisely what it needs to nurture itself even while detoxifying.

Set a pretty table, relax, and take your time when breaking the fast. You will want to be conscious of the way you feel after every bite. Notice the changes that have taken place in the last few days. Does your stomach seem smaller? Don't stuff yourself. Chew your food well and stop eating the instant you no longer feel hungry. Your digestive system is at its most sensitive. Respect the signals it sends you. Are you craving processed or sugary foods? You may have dredged up some toxins that are stimulating those cravings. Don't give in. One of my clients thought she could sneak in just a mouthful or two of white carbs after her fast, and she became extremely ill.

A general rule for breaking a fast is that for every day that you fasted, you should spend half that time breaking the fast. So if you fasted for three days, you'll spend a day and a half gently easing out of it. If you fasted for four days, you'll spend two days breaking it, and so on. I recommend that you wait until you have completely eased out of the fast before reintroducing the Green Meal Shake or any other sweet foods to your diet.

The day after the fast, I ate more salad than I thought I could eat in a day! It gave me so much energy! I felt lighter. After this cleanse, my skin cleared up, I lost weight, my asthma lightened, and my bloating and intestinal problems stopped. I learned what is necessary to have a healthy diet and body. Thanks, Karyn. —T. C.

Your body is constantly rebuilding itself from the cellular level up. That means you literally become what you eat. Feed yourself with delicious, raw food fresh from the earth, and you will rebuild your body on a foundation laid by Mother Nature herself.

As you break your fast, don't sweat any final cleansing symptoms that come your way. You may, for instance, find your sleep patterns have been disturbed. You may not feel tired until four in the morning. And even after falling asleep so late, you may rise at the crack of dawn. Or you may not have a bowel movement for several days following the cleanse and fast. You may experience flatulence or even a bit of nausea. Just remind yourself that these are signs of your transformation, then let these little changes go. You are alive and healthier than ever. Lucky you!

REBALANCE WITH BREATH WORK

As we have said, the fast works its magic on two planes: the physical and the spiritual. As your body adjusts after the fast, you may want to experiment with some bodywork to help incorporate the physical and spiritual benefits into one vital channel of living energy. I suggest breath work. Slowing the breath can aid your health and well-being. After all, tortoises and elephants, two of the longest-living animals in the wild, are also among the slowest breathers.

This Sufi technique that I learned in India will pull the cleansing oxygen through your body to detox your internal organs, relax you, and make your body and mind work as one. To begin, assume a meditative position. I suggest sitting on large, comfortable pillows on the floor. Make sure your environment is quiet and dimly lit. Make yourself comfortable, close your eyes, and open your palms. Inhale slowly through your nose, filling your lungs for five counts. Hold the breath in for five counts, then exhale through your nose for five counts. Continue the breathing until it becomes rhythmic and natural.

When you have adapted to this breathing pattern, begin a healing visualization. Think, for instance, of the color gold. Consider the warmth and illumination that this color represents. Imagine yourself bathed in a field of gold, completely swaddled in its life-giving presence. With each breath, pull this presence inside you. Let it energize you like the sun, the source of all. Now visualize yourself in meditation, rooted to the place you now sit. Your roots ground you to the source of all. You are breathing in the light energy that surrounds you. As you breathe, release your shoulders, your back muscles, and any tension in your body. Now exhale, relax, and concentrate on the breath. Repeat the visualization with the colors green, red, white, and blue.

This technique rapidly delivers oxygen to the cells. Do it while you are sitting in traffic and you will be transported to a place of calm clarity. Use it for a few days and you will be suffused with well-being. Use it for a week and you will do it forever. Your health is within your power. Your body has shown you how to use that power wisely.

WEEK 3: FREQUENTLY ASKED QUESTIONS

Q: Are there any medical conditions that can make fasting hazardous?

A: Fasting is usually not dangerous, especially when you have carefully prepared your body for it as we have during this program. However, for people who have hypoglycemia or insulin-dependent diabetes, or those who have recently had major surgery, fasting should only be undertaken with a physician's supervision. If you have any of these conditions or are taking any medications, please consult a qualified health-care professional before beginning a fast.

Q: I became very emotional during the fast. Is that common?

A: Fasting switches the body's normal function to purge mode. As toxins are released, emotions surface. These are emotions that need to be released.

Q: Will fasting provide me with enough vitamins and minerals?

A: Your body is a vast storehouse of nutrients. You can live on what your body has stored for much longer than the duration of this fast. Moreover, you will be

getting more than the recommended daily allowance of vitamins and minerals in the kamut water, rejuvelac, and wheatgrass juice you will be drinking. Not only will you be suitably nourished, you will also be getting more vitamins than you would from a burger and fries.

TABLE 3. Week 3 protocol summary

During Week 3, the focus is on the fast.

FOOD/PRODUCT	INSTRUCTIONS	TIMING	BENEFITS
Fast	On the days that you fast, consume liquids only: ▪ spirulina water (2 to 4 ounces daily) ▪ fresh vegetable juice (containing carrots, celery, collard greens, cucumber, kale, parsley, and spinach) ▪ rejuvelac ▪ kamut water ▪ purified water with OxyKare ▪ wheatgrass juice (2 to 4 ounces daily) Do **not** consume the following during your fast: ▪ fenugreek seed capsules ▪ Energy Soup ▪ fruit juice ▪ Green Meal Shake ▪ psyllium and detox clay **Note:** It is essential that you continue daily colonics or enemas (followed by implants) during your fast.	Fast for 3 or more consecutive days.	Fasting is the best means of cleansing and detoxification.
Oil of oregano	Take a dropperful once or twice a day.	Take anytime on the days that you are fasting.	Oil of oregano is antibacterial, antimicrobial, and combats yeast.
Systemic enzymes	Take 3 capsules 2 times a day.	Anytime on days you are fasting. At other times, always on an empty stomach.	Reduces inflammation and strengthens the immune system.
Breaking the fast	Continue eating only raw food, including: ▪ Energy Soup ▪ Green Meal Shake ▪ light salads ▪ sprout salads ▪ pâtés	Reintroduce raw foods slowly and carefully as needed to satisfy your hunger.	After a fast, the body has become unused to digesting food. Proceed with patience, or the good of the fast will be undone.

TABLE 4. Optional for Week 3

PRODUCT	INSTRUCTIONS	TIMING	BENEFITS
Probiotics (Ultra Flora)	Take 3 capsules 2 times a day.	Take one dose anytime during the day; take the other after your daily enema or colonic.	Probiotics populate and promote the growth of beneficial bacteria in the small and large intestines.
Digestive enzymes	Take with your fresh vegetable juice.	Take anytime.	Digestive enzymes break down food so that nutrients quickly pass through the intestinal walls, circulate through the bloodstream, and nourish the body's cells.
Coconut water	Drink any amount desired.	Drink anytime. Can be used as a chaser after drinking wheatgrass juice.	Coconut water helps balance electrolytes and rehydrates.

TABLE 5. Other considerations for Week 3

THERAPY	INSTRUCTIONS	TIMING	BENEFITS
Self-care	Avoid smoke-filled rooms, stressful situations, skin products that contain chemicals, and strenuous workouts. Instead, do gentle yoga or use a mini trampoline for heel lifts, running, or jumping.	Try to do some form of self-care every day of the fast.	Your body and emotions are vulnerable during a fast. It is important to take good care of yourself.
Body care	Brush your skin, always brushing toward the heart, when it is dry or when you are in the sauna. Bathe in 1 to 3 pounds of sea salt to remove toxins. Instead of lotion, moisturize with sesame oil during your fast and with olive oil after your fast.	Try to do some form of body care every day.	These actions help the body rid itself of toxins and wastes.
Healing breath work	See page 86 for detailed instructions for rhythmic breathing and visualization.	Try to do healing breath work every day.	Breath work enhances well-being and reduces stress levels.

TESTIMONIALS

During Week 4 of my classes in Chicago, many students stand in front of the room and share their experience with me and their fellow detoxers. As a group we laugh, we cry, we cheer each other on. Other students will write or email their comments to me later. These testimonials are the true energy behind this program. I am just one person who had my life changed by the powerful effects of raw food and detoxification. It is the thousands of people who have taken this journey with me who make it a movement. The people who shared their testimonials are my fellow teachers; they are your guides and support system. I would love it if you would also become a teacher and share your experience by emailing me at karyninfo@karynraw.com. Miracles—small, large, and anywhere in between—are welcome. Your stories are what keep me going day after day. They are what drive me to grow my business and to continue spreading this message to as many people who care to listen. I am deeply grateful for your contribution.

Even though I have been a vegetarian for five years, this cleanse has taught me how to listen to my bodily responses and know why they are happening.

—A. N.

After working with Karyn, my life has opened and transformed in new and profound directions. Karyn exudes an attitude of contribution, not competition, in her philosophy of optimal health. Modern medicine and science have yet to recognize the miracles of those who have experienced Karyn's work in holistic health.

—S. B.

This has been a spiritual awakening for me. After 28 days, I'm happy to say I found another person inside this body.

—F. G.

The detox class has been just as much a spiritual journey as a physical one.

—B. B.

celebration

DAYS 22 TO 28

Twenty-one days and countless bottles of rejuvelac later, you have arrived at Week 4. Sure, your path might not have been precisely straight and narrow. Change is very difficult, and old habits are hard to break. For all its ups and downs, twists and turns, this journey has been entirely your own—an adventure that led you along the pathway to healing. Regardless of what detours you took, your trip has turned out exactly right. And that is something to celebrate!

You have learned a lot in the last three weeks. You have learned, for example, that your body is the repository of nature's awesome wisdom, and that this wisdom can guide your life and transform your awareness. You've learned that healing is never the result of a magic shot or pill. It is what happens when your inborn emotional, mental, and physical energies align into one powerful, inextinguishable life force. You have also learned what it means to live and fuel your body as God intended. And, most importantly, it is my hope that you have fallen in love with yourself again.

Cleansing can be a test, but it is never a contest. It is a winding path that delivers us to the heart of our challenges, to the depths of despair, and to the launch site of miracles—sometimes all in the same week! Somehow, along the way, we arrive at the certain knowledge that our well-being is within our control.

Week 4 at a Glance

Continue the following:

- 100 percent raw diet
- chlorella tablets
- Green Meal Shake
- kamut water
- rejuvelac
- spirulina water
- wheatgrass juice

The following are **optional**:

- fenugreek seed capsules
- OxyKare in 32 ounces of purified water
- psyllium and detox clay

For a detailed summary of the Week 4 cleansing protocol, see pages 101–103.

WEEK 4: WHAT CONTINUES

Congratulations! You've made it to Week 4. I'm sure you feel a huge sense of accomplishment. I'm also sure you are ready to get back to reality. We can't be in cleansing mode forever, after all. But before you hang up your detox hat, I'm going to ask one more thing of you. It is only Day 22, after all!

For this final week of your cleansing program, I want you to continue eating only 100 percent raw foods. You have worked hard, remained determined, and fought through your cleansing reactions. This is the chance to seal in your results and ensure that the wonderful healing effects of your detox resonate throughout your body. So, please, for just one more week, continue to feed your body the bountiful nourishment that is naturally occurring on this earth. You'll be glad you did.

If you are still fasting, you will want to stay 100 percent raw for one week after completing your fast. You can undo all the benefits of your fast by returning too quickly to eating cooked foods and, even worse, animal-based foods.

In addition, during Week 4 you can continue the drinks and supplements that have worked for you during the preceding weeks. These include the Green Meal Shake, chlorella tablets, kamut water, rejuvelac, spirulina water, and wheatgrass juice.

WEEK 4 AND BEYOND: WHAT'S OPTIONAL

Supplementing with fenugreek seed capsules is optional for up to two months after the cleanse. Unless you've been dealing with sugar, alcohol, or drug addiction, you can reduce your daily dosage of fenugreek. When I am stressed and hit the sugar (that's when I buy mangoes by the case!), I always reach for fenugreek. It helps me to control my impulses before I do any real damage.

If fenugreek is what stands between you and your next sugar binge, by all means, continue to pop it. Just figure out how much of the herb feels right for you. Some people take up to four capsules twice a day with great results. You can also continue to use fenugreek water in your enema bucket for as long as you need to remove excess mucus. Just bear in mind that most herbal remedies begin to lose their effect after they have been taken continuously for three months. Some can even turn on you. So give yourself a short break between courses of herbal therapies. That way your supplements will do you the most good from cleanse to cleanse.

After the cleanse, you are free to eliminate the psyllium and detox clay from your daily regimen unless you feel you have an excess of candida in your system. As we've seen, candida can play havoc with your health. There's no better time than immediately following a cleanse to get a troublesome case in check. If your candida didn't end with the cleanse, continue the psyllium and detox clay treat-

ments for another thirty days. I also recommend that you take oil of oregano, colloidal silver, or grapefruit seed extract twice a day. All are natural antibiotics and effective digestive tract cleansers. They will work in conjunction with the psyllium to clear away the debris that feeds yeast.

Psyllium and detox clay are extremely powerful drawing agents. Therefore, I suggest that you continue these treatments for a maximum of three months. As for the psyllium and oil of oregano combination, adjust it until you find the right dose for your body. If the cleansing seems a bit strong, try taking the oil of oregano, colloidal silver, or grapefruit seed extract only once a day.

AFTER YOUR CLEANSE

As I said earlier, I recommend doing a full cleanse four times a year. Each detox functions like a vehicle that picks us up where we are and delivers us to a new destination. Needless to say, it is important that you realistically evaluate your physical condition, your needs, your cravings, and your goals immediately after this cleanse. This will help you to maintain the wonderful changes you've already made. It also provides you with a milestone for the future, so you can better gauge just how much closer each subsequent cleanse brings you to your ultimate goal.

In between cleanses, you can rely on aspects of your cleansing program to keep you in optimal health. Keep the program alive by maintaining what is meaningful to you. If you've found a menu of revitalizing foods that work for you, you're onto something. It's like they say: whatever works!

I entered Karyn's class with high expectations, and I did not believe they would be met. I wanted better overall health, an awareness of what foods would energize my body, increased discipline with food and exercise, knowledge of alternative food and exercise, weight loss (or at least inches off everything except my height and bust) and, most importantly, normal and regular elimination. A bit much, I would say. At best, I expected to achieve knowledge, not results. Yet I have surpassed all of my expectations! What I have not been able to do in four years, I did in weeks. This class has given me knowledge for a lifetime. It has been an unbelievable and valuable journey. —C. M.

Keep What Works

You might decide, for instance, to become a vegetarian or a vegan. You might try to maintain a diet that is 60 percent raw. Or you might opt to eat raw meals all week and then go back to cooked meals on weekends. Whatever you decide, be sure to set a comfortable goal for yourself. Most people are trying to nourish themselves while eating diets that are only 5 percent raw. Anything you do beyond that is a plus.

Many of the drinks and supplements you used during your cleanse can be continued indefinitely. These include the Green Meal Shake, rejuvelac, wheatgrass juice, kamut, spirulina water, and chlorella tablets. I can't tell you how many cleansing alumni have made the Green Meal Shake a mainstay of their post-cleanse diet. If, over time, the drink gets too sweet for you, eliminate the banana or add more rejuvelac. You can even make it in big batches and store it in glass containers in the refrigerator.

I used to be caught up in the marketing of "fat free." If there was no fat, it had to be good for you. I didn't even think about the sugar or preservatives in all these foods. I initially took Karyn's class because I had food poisoning from meat. I knew I had to take control and break old habits. Going through the class, I noticed how much food controls my moods. After this class, the energy level I have is incredible. And I am integrating the information I received from Karyn into my everyday life. It's not a diet; it's a way of life. —G.

Speaking of products that work—OxyKare and Green Kamut Powder are two products that stave off yeast imbalances and will forever be in my cupboard. Choose the amount of Green Kamut Powder that feels right to you. This should be between 1 and 4 tablespoons in 16 to 32 ounces of purified water. To me, this is a deeply satisfying drink that fortifies my feeling of balance. It may be something you want to carry with you on your journey as well. I've been drinking one capful of OxyKare in 32 ounces of purified water fairly regularly for the past thirty years. OxyKare is powerful, though, so give your body periodic breaks from taking it.

Mini Fasts

Celebrate your new awareness with some new traditions. A cleanse reminds you that the food you eat today may be what's eating you tomorrow! In order to maintain your focus on healthful eating, you might want to set aside one day a week for fasting. As we have seen, fasts can range in intensity from total abstinence from solid food to a diet limited to certain types of foods, such as juices or Energy Soup. If you have gone back to eating animal products, fasting is particularly important. Whether you define your fast as one day of every week when you eat only raw food or a twenty-four-hour period during which you restrict yourself to liquids, fasting as a part of your weekly regimen reaffirms your body's memory of the cleansing experience and retains your focus on self-nurturance.

Colonic Irrigation

Enemas are certainly beneficial. However, if it's at all possible, I suggest you have a series of ten colonics twice a year. As anyone who has tried both enemas and colonics will certainly attest, colonics are the most gentle, effective way to

loosen and sweep away impacted fecal matter and plaque. Almost everyone I know who has tried colonics after having enemas says that hydrotherapy makes an incredible difference.

In addition to regular "clean outs," there are specific circumstances that warrant hydrotherapy. If you've been away on vacation, particularly to an exotic locale where you've been eating food that is out of the ordinary, follow up with a series of colonics. If you are juice fasting one day a week and want to get the most out of your fast, you might want to do an enema and an implant. The one thing I don't recommend, though, is doing an enema or colonic without following up with an implant. An implant replaces the colonic flora you have flushed from the digestive tract. It also helps to maintain your system's balance so you will never become addicted to hydrotherapy or dependent on flushing to keep the waste moving.

Of course, you can't expect to have a normal bowel movement if you've been fasting and taking enemas. The wastes will simply not collect the same way. But if you are careful to follow hydrotherapy with an implant, your bowels will respond appropriately when you resume your normal eating pattern.

Seek Support

Your new lifestyle may feel challenging at times. You may be tempted to do the easy thing rather than the right one. That's why I suggest that you make a conscious effort to remind yourself of the wonderful benefits you've reaped from this cleanse by keeping in touch with your cleansing buddy, treating yourself to a meal at a raw-food restaurant, participating in a support group, or seeking support from books or online.

Raw cuisine is at the height of its popularity right now. If you can't treat yourself to a great meal at a raw-food restaurant, host a potluck dinner and serve your favorite raw dishes. I encourage you to start your own support group or at least stay in touch with your fasting buddy. When your buddy is not available, seek support from books or the many active and informative raw-food lifestyle websites, where you can find everything from recipes to seminar schedules to emotional sustenance.

On those days when the chips are down (or on their way down the hatch!), take a moment to reread your cleansing journal. Recall what you felt like when you were pushing the toxins out of your body. Ask yourself, do you feel that way now? At no time are you closer to your ideal health than immediately after

Other differences [in me since my cleanse]: I purchased a wheatgrass juicer and juice at home now. I bought a raw-food recipe book. I felt totally fine and normal and proud when people asked me what I was doing and why. I encouraged friends to join me, and they did! I released more and more emotionally—and more of my old lifestyle. I thank the universe for bringing me to Karyn. —T. T.

a cleanse. Take the steps necessary to stay close to that feeling and you can add years to your life—and life to your years.

Stay Sane When Snacking

People let go of their cravings when they're ready and not a moment before. For example, I passed up meat, chucked out the chicken, and even gave ice cream the heave ho, but I had a very hard time giving up popcorn. In fact, I was a popcorn-eating raw foodist for years. Since it was important that I do something to diminish the negative effects of my food addiction, I started sprinkling my popcorn with spirulina and papayazyme to make it easier to digest until the day I could give it up altogether.

Nothing provides a better boost than spirulina. Tossed in a salad or soup, spirulina flakes add flavor while calming those hunger pangs. Because it's convenient to use and keep, spirulina is a snack-time staple that's easy to take wherever you go. Keep it within reach and you'll always have something nearby to nosh on without having to resort to processed, sugary, or fatty alternatives.

I highly encourage you to incorporate at least one or two greens into your daily life. Inevitably, someone always asks me which green is the absolute best. My answer? The best green is the one that you will eat or drink consistently.

Reconsider Animal Products

I'm a realist. I know that you may not become vegan or even vegetarian for the rest of your life. If you go back to eating animal-based foods, you may want to try organic and free-range products, even though they are not perfect options. A smart choice may be to visit farmers' markets and get to know your local farmers. If you feel that you must eat animal-based foods, learn where they really come from. And be sure to take at least four to five digestive enzymes before eating a meal that contains animal products to help your body break them down.

If you do make the choice to stay vegan, I encourage you to supplement with vitamin B_{12}. Although this nutrient is commonly misunderstood, it has become a frequent argument against a solely plant-based diet. A

I came to this program because I have a severe case of candida. My condition stems from using massive doses of antibiotics to treat a bone infection. [Since the cleanse], I feel much better. Many of my symptoms have improved. My feet and nails have always been full of fungus. Since this detox, my feet feel so much better. Also, my legs were heavy and painful, and my lymph nodes were sore to the touch. This has also improved. Emotionally, I feel much better. I feel more grounded, more centered, and more complete. Some days I actually feel wonderful. It was a great program. —**M.**

vitamin B_{12} deficiency is just as likely to occur in meat eaters as it is in vegans because of a lack of the intrinsic factor that enables the body to absorb it. While studies have shown that vitamin B_{12} can be obtained by eating certain animal-based foods, research has not established a reliable source of B_{12} in plant foods. I have been a vegan for over thirty years and rarely supplement with B_{12}. I believe that the fermented foods, like sauerkraut and rejuvelac, in my diet are to credit. However, there is no conclusive data to prove this and the harmful, long-term effects of a B_{12} deficiency can be difficult or impossible to reverse. Therefore, I recommend that all vegans take at least 10 micrograms of vitamin B_{12} daily, and that everyone, regardless of dietary preference, supplement with B_{12}.

If you are willing to avoid one animal food consistently after your cleanse, let it be dairy. Because most cow's milk is so tainted by antibiotics, growth hormones, and steroids, dairy products are extremely mucus-producing and certainly toxic. Even raw and organic dairy products, which are touted by some alternative-health practitioners, are far from being ideal fuels for our bodies.

Cancer and heart disease aren't just out there picking and choosing among us. These diseases are by-products of the toxins we call "food." In the 1800s, it was the wealthy that almost exclusively had coronary thrombosis and heart disease because they could afford to eat so much meat. Today, many people include meat or dairy in every meal. If you have learned anything over the last 28 days, it is that mucus prevents the body from taking in nutrients. These foods produce mucus, among many other harmful effects.

Even if you eat completely raw all week but eat just a little dairy on the weekend, it will eventually produce enough plaque in your digestive system to block the absorption of essential nutrients. If you like the creaminess of dairy, there are many wonderful dairy alternatives in grocery stores these days. Soy and rice products are probably the most readily available. However, keep in mind that processed soy in large quantities can be quite mucus forming, and I believe this is one of the reasons there are so many unhealthy vegetarians and vegans out there. While soy can be a good bridge food for those who are transitioning away from meat and dairy, products made from almonds, coconut, and hemp are much better choices.

Be Kind to Your Skin

Skin care isn't usually a crucial topic for me when I teach a cleansing seminar because I want detoxers to concentrate on changing their skin from within. Age lines will diminish naturally with consistent good eating. But since the skin is an important excretory organ, you should do what you can to help it move toxins out through the pores so they can be washed away.

Waste materials don't just hide in the digestive tract; they also lurk in the layers of tissue below the epidermis. But relief is within reach. Detox clay, the same volcanic ash you've used to pull impurities from the intestines, also works as a powerful, fragrance-free, and additive-free drawing agent on the skin. Liquid detox clay can be applied directly to the skin. If you are using powdered detox clay, simply mix it with plain water to make a paste. As it dries, it will draw out poison and tighten the pores.

If you have mature skin or need to exfoliate, I recommend a scrub or clay mask. These products, which I use once or twice every week, slough off dead skin cells to reveal noticeably clearer, brighter skin—even for women in menopause who need to make up for sluggish cell turnover. These treatments are totally optional, of course, but they do make skin glow, augmenting the brightness you have already taken on as a result of the cleanse.

DON'T FORGET WHAT YOU KNOW

Knowing how to cleanse when you need to, for as long as you need to, can be your protective shield against all the negativity in the world. We are subject to many negative factors that influence the way we live, think, and nurture ourselves. Therefore, it is important that we remember to use our protective shield when we need to.

I frequently use cleansing techniques when I need to recover from unhealthful influences. For example, my husband and I were invited to a business-related party, so we had no choice but to attend. We decided to get there early so we could leave early. We arrived at eight thirty sharp, left our car with the valet, and went in.

The party was held in a beautiful, spacious home, but by nine thirty it was bursting at the seams with at least 150 guests. Because many of them were from countries where cigarette smoking is still an accepted practice, the air was increasingly cloudy and thick. By now you realize that although I am devoted to living the purest lifestyle possible, I'm also a realist. I am used to living in a polluted world. Nevertheless, cigarette smoke is one toxin that has a serious effect on my sinuses and lungs, making me immediately fatigued.

As casually as possible, I worked my way over to a window and opened it a crack. A man came over to engage me in conversation. We chatted about forty-five seconds before he felt a draft and shut the window. By the time dinner—a

I Can't Go a Day Without . . .

During Week 4 of the cleanse, someone inevitably asks me what my average day is like: what food I eat, what supplements I take, what exercises I do. While I insist that you listen to your body and create a routine that is practical and nurturing for you, I am happy to share my daily essentials as an example. But remember, these essentials have been on my list for years. I didn't go from A to Z overnight, and you shouldn't expect to either.

KARYN'S DAILY ESSENTIALS

- prayer and meditation
- chlorella, 12 to 24 tablets
- coconut oil, 2 tablespoons
- coenzyme Q10, 200 milligrams
- digestive enzymes with every meal
- exercise on my rebounder (mini trampoline), 15 minutes
- Karyn's Kare Green Kamut Powder, 2 to 4 tablespoons in water
- Karyn's Kare Green Meal Shake
- Karyn's Kare Green Living Fiber, 4 to 6 capsules
- Karyn's Kare OxyKare Vitamin O, 1 capful in 32 ounces purified water
- Karyn's Kare Systemic Enzymes
- rejuvelac with aloe, 1 glass
- some form of fermented food, such as sauerkraut or Cashew Sour Cream (page 114)
- spirulina, 1 to 2 tablespoons in a smoothie or a salad
- spirulina water, 2 to 4 ounces
- vitamin C, 800 milligrams
- vitamin D_3, 2,000 IU
- wheatgrass juice, 2 to 4 ounces
- yoga, 30 minutes
- young green coconut water, 1 to 2 ounces

Vitamin D supplementation, which I list above but have not mentioned earlier in the book, is essential. Experts estimate that 70 to 90 percent of North Americans don't get enough vitamin D. Sunshine and supplements are excellent sources. Although some foods, such as milk, are fortified with vitamin D, they generally do not provide enough to significantly improve health. And as we know, milk is an unnatural and unhealthful food for people.

For information about how to order products, including the Karyn's Kare line of supplements, see Resources, page 119.

cooked-food buffet featuring an enormous ham leg—was served, the atmosphere was beginning to get to my husband too. We decided to make our escape but were unsuccessful. The valet informed us that, since we had been among the first to arrive, our car was now trapped in an enormous, stationary traffic jam of parked cars. Worse, while we waited and the valet began to reshuffle the vehicles, our host noticed us loitering on the lawn. "You're not leaving, are you?" he called to us. "Why don't you come back in? We're just about to break out the cognac!"

So there we were, trapped in a virtual smokestack until one thirty. Even after I was out of the fray, the effects of the night went on and on. Two hours after going to bed, I was jolted awake by heart palpitations. I felt like I was drowning in the mucus

that my body had produced to protect itself from the toxins. But I knew exactly what to do. I immediately began a cleanse to restore my body to its natural balance.

A FINAL WORD

I always like to ask new detoxers what brought them to my door. On the night before Day 1 of the program, most of the newbies tell me the same thing: they have come to my class to lose weight. By Day 7, their priorities have changed dramatically.

Disease is usually easy to identify. It has distinct and often disturbing symptoms. It disrupts our lives. But "dis-ease" is much more subtle. While serious illness hits us in the face like a bucket of water, dis-ease envelops us gradually, like a slow-rolling fog. Now, most of us don't feel miserably sick all the time, but we don't feel that great either. When somebody asks us how we are, we say we're fine because, although we have aches and pains and digestive problems and insomnia and maybe a little touch of arthritis or sinus headaches or itchy skin or whatever else, we're not really sick. Or are we? On Day 1 of the cleanse, we don't think so. But by Day 7, when the fog has finally begun to lift, things don't look the same to us anymore. We not only realize that we have been sick, but we also see for the first time that *we* have made ourselves sick. Suddenly we don't see our weight as the problem anymore. Rather, we view it as just another symptom. That is when we start healing— mentally, emotionally, and physically.

When the fog lifted for me more than thirty-five years ago, I stopped feeling like a victim of my genes. I began to feel, for the first time in my life, that I was in control of the wonderful body God gave me to live in. If, at the end of this experience, you feel the same, then you have a great deal to celebrate. You no longer need to fear our toxic environment or foods. You are in control of what goes into your body. You no longer need to fear illness, despite your genes or predispositions. You know how to do the right thing for your health and longevity. Most of all, you no longer need to fear your lack of willpower or weakness for certain foods or any other tendency people characterize as "failure."

In the last 28 exciting, transformative days, you have seen that if you fall off the wagon, if you are exposed to toxins, if you eat meat or dairy, you can detoxify every system of your body and begin again. God, in His or Her wisdom, has provided us with a body that constantly renews itself. All you need to do to bring that renewal to fruition is to align your thinking with what is natural, vital, and good. Focus your mind on all that is pure and alive and bursting with energy, and the rest of you will surely follow.

In these 28 short days, you have broken down the layers of habit and self-deception to reveal the essential truth we are all born with. You have tapped

into your own infallible intuition. Now you must find a way to live what you know to be true. Choose a reasonable goal. Do what you can to maintain the beneficial changes you've made but bear in mind that perfection is not a requirement. You've got all the chances you need to get it right. You may not be able to commit to detoxing multiple times a year in the beginning of your journey. But if you can commit to just picking up and reading this book a few times a year, you will be able to keep it in practice. Find ways to constantly remind yourself of the powerful life changes you've created, and you will never be far from the truth.

Most of all, I hope that you will share what you have learned during this process. Sharing what I have learned, sharing the lessons my body continues to teach me every day, is truly the joy of my life. It will be the same for you, I know. What you have come to know about the synergy between inner healing and vital, radiant beauty will resonate with others and help them find their way.

I also hope that you will share your ongoing journey with me. Please feel free to email me at karyninfo@karynraw.com. I'd love to hear about your challenges and your miracles.

I'll leave you with this reminder: *If you don't take care of your body—the most magnificent machine you'll ever be given—where are you going to live?*

I wish you love, peace, and health.

TABLE 6. Week 4 protocol summary

This summary covers what you should continue through Week 4 and the end of your cleanse. It also provides information about what you can do beyond the cleanse.

FOOD/SUPPLEMENT	WEEK 4 AND GOING FORWARD	MORE INFORMATION	BENEFITS
Raw diet	Continue eating only raw foods for one week after breaking your fast. You can maintain your raw diet indefinitely.	See raw-food recipe books in Resources (page 119) or experiment with making your own raw-food recipes.	Eating a raw diet will keep your body alkalized and help you sustain and continue weight loss. A raw diet is rich in minerals and nutrients for optimal health.
Green Meal Shake	Use during Week 4; can be continued indefinitely.	Follow the recipe (page 118) or modify the ingredients to keep it interesting.	The Green Meal Shake is a nutrient-dense raw superfood that is easy for your body to digest. It improves metabolism and calcium absorption.

(continued)

TABLE 6. Continued

FOOD/SUPPLEMENT	WEEK 4 AND GOING FORWARD	MORE INFORMATION	BENEFITS
Rejuvelac	Use during Week 4; can be continued indefinitely.	Drink as much as you like. Rejuvelac can replace water.	Rejuvelac is good for stress and helps clean the intestinal tract by loosening mucus. It contains B vitamins, enzymes, and protein. It is a nondairy source of the beneficial bacteria lactobacillus.
Spirulina water	Use during Week 4; can be continued indefinitely.	Use any desired amount.	Spirulina provides balanced, whole superfood nutrition that is easily digested and absorbed for vigor and health.
Wheatgrass juice	Use during Week 4; can be continued indefinitely.	Use any desired amount.	Wheatgrass juice is an excellent source of nutrients and enzymes that strengthen the digestive system and combat toxicity.
Chlorella tablets	Use during Week 4; can be continued indefinitely.	Larger doses can be used as a main protein source in a vegan diet.	Chlorella strengthens the digestive system and combats heavy metal and environmental toxicity.
Fenugreek seed capsules	Optional during Week 4. Do not take for more than 3 consecutive months.	Take a break for 4 to 6 weeks before resuming use.	Fenugreek seed capsules balance blood sugar levels and clean the lymphatic system. As with any herb, fenugreek is meant to be used temporarily. Continued use without a break could cause negative side effects.
Psyllium and detox clay	Optional for Week 4. Do not take more than 3 consecutive months.	Take a break for 4 to 6 weeks before resuming use. Allow your body to work on its own.	The psyllium-detox clay cocktail cleanses mucus-forming toxic waste from the colon.
Fresh vegetable juice	Can be continued indefinitely.	Try different juice combinations.	Fresh vegetable juice is alkalizing and provides concentrated vitamins and minerals.
Kamut water	Can be continued indefinitely.	Use any amount desired.	Kamut is alkalizing and promotes digestive health and regularity.
OxyKare	Take for 3 to 6 months and then take a break from it.	Never more than one capful in 32 ounces of purified water.	OxyKare detoxifies cells and combats yeast. Best to use on a cleanse or as a healing agent against common colds, flus, and infections.

TABLE 6. Continued

FOOD/SUPPLEMENT	WEEK 4 AND GOING FORWARD	MORE INFORMATION	BENEFITS
Digestive enzymes	Can be continued indefinitely. Take with each meal.	Vary amount based on desired results.	Digestive enzymes break down food so that nutrients quickly pass through the intestinal walls, circulate through the bloodstream, and nourish the body's cells.
Systemic enzymes	Can be continued indefinitely. Take on an empty stomach.	Vary amount based on desired results.	Great to boost your immune system and to support your body when faced with larger medical challenges.
Energy Soup	Choose this nutritious meal anytime.	Modify the recipe to keep it interesting.	Energy Soup is easy to digest. It is an excellent source of healthful fats, nutrients, and vitamins.
Coconut oil	Can be continued indefinitely. Use internally and topically.	Use in smoothies and recipes.	Coconut oil promotes skin health; combats yeast, parasites, and fungus; and supports heart and brain health.
Oil of oregano	Take when necessary, but do not take every day indefinitely.	When using oil of oregano (or any natural antibiotic), make sure you are replenishing with probiotics.	Oil of oregano is great for combating colds, flu, headache, infection, stomachache, yeast, and many ailments.
Enemas, colonics, and implants	A series of colonics or enemas a few times a year can be highly beneficial. Do not continue indefinitely. Allow your body to work on its own.	Use during a cleanse or when cleansing symptoms arise. An implant should be done following every colonic or enema.	Enemas and colonics help relieve headaches, stomachaches, and other symptoms. They also improve colon health and nutrient absorption.

Having previously eaten anything I desired made switching to a raw diet pretty difficult, but I followed the program to a T, and I've never felt better. —E. C.

Although I was a vegetarian before I started the detox, I still did not eat well. I ate too much food and a lot of sweets, and I did not really feel that I had any control over my eating habits. I felt sluggish, had trouble concentrating, was often tired, and had little energy. I knew that many of my problems were related to my diet. Karyn's detoxification program was one of my best decisions. Not only have I done something wonderful for my body, but I also feel better, have lost weight, and finally feel in control of my nutrition and many other aspects my life. —A. C.

I'm glad I did this. Every step has been a journey. This is just the beginning for me. The way I feel and look has no price tag! —H. H.

I am so glad that Karyn has developed a program where weight loss is not the focus but a secondary advantage. It is also great that she treats health as a complete system, with mind, body, and spirit working in harmony as the goal. As a result of the program, I look at what I put into my body differently, and I reflect on which experiences I wish to put into my life. —L. H.

This was my first class with Karyn, and I will never be the same. I see a long, wonderful road ahead, leading me toward being as well as possible. —E. N.

recipes FOR THE CLEANSE

I have created hundreds of recipes over the years in my restaurant and my personal life. There are endless possibilities to keep a raw diet interesting and satisfying so that it's a sustainable, long-term choice for you. I've included a few recipes here to support you during the cleanse.

None of these require equipment beyond a food processor or blender. However, as you begin to incorporate more raw foods into your life, you may want to acquire some of the other "essential" equipment used in raw-food preparation. Visit my website, www.karynraw.com, for further information and to order dehydrators, juicers, and more.

I am already looking forward to my next cleanse. Now I know I will do it four times a year. I realize that this is a process, and I cannot reverse my life overnight. My ultimate goal is to become 100 percent raw, and I feel that I am well on my way. A huge thank you to Karyn. —J. L.

Rejuvelac

Rejuvelac is rich in B vitamins and protein, and because it is fermented, it contains beneficial bacteria and active enzymes. Drink it straight, as a beverage, or use it in recipes, such as Green Meal Shake (page 118) or Dr. Wigmore's Energy Soup (page 112).

2 cups wheat berries

10 cups purified water

Soak the wheat berries in 4 cups of the water for 24 hours.

Drain and rinse the wheat berries in a large mesh colander and set aside for 24 hours at room temperature. During this time, the wheat berries will sprout (small white "tails" will appear). If the wheat berries do not sprout after 24 hours, let them sit for a few more hours until they do.

Transfer the wheat berries to a food processor or blender and process until smooth. Put the ground wheat berries into a clean glass jar or large glass container and add the remaining 6 cups of water. Cover the jar with cheesecloth or a mesh screen to allow oxygen to get into the mixture (secure with string or a rubber band). Let ferment at room temperature for at least 48 hours. The longer the Rejuvelac ferments, the stronger the it will be.

Strain the Rejuvelac into clean glass jars and cover tightly. Stored in the refrigerator, Rejuvelac will keep for 4 weeks.

TIP: If you don't drink all the Rejuvelac before it spoils, it's great for watering plants.

Nut Milk

Soaked nuts and seeds can be used to make tasty alternatives to dairy milk and cheeses. Nut Milk is a common ingredient in many raw recipes.

1 cup raw almonds or other raw nuts or seeds

6 cups purified water

1 to 2 tablespoons agave nectar or other sweetener

$1/2$ teaspoon vanilla extract

Soak the almonds in 3 cups of the water for 8 to 12 hours.

Drain and rinse the almonds. Transfer the almonds to a blender and add the remaining 3 cups of water. Process on high speed for 30 seconds, or until the liquid is smooth. Strain into a clean glass jar through a nut-milk bag, a sieve lined with cheesecloth, or a clean knee-high stocking. Whisk in the agave nectar and vanilla extract. Stored in a sealed glass jar in the refrigerator, Nut Milk will keep for 5 to 7 days.

TIPS

- If you have a twin-gear juicer, run the blended mixture through the juicer using the vegetable screen; this will provide the smoothest Nut Milk possible. Save the pulp to add to other recipes.

- If you are diabetic or watching your sugar intake, stevia is a good alternative to agave nectar or other sweeteners. Stevia is very sweet, so only a small amount is needed. Follow the directions on the stevia package and sweeten to taste.

Green Meal Shake

This delicious shake makes a satisfying raw breakfast or snack that will keep you feeling full and balanced for hours. It is rich in calcium, essential fatty acids, fiber, minerals, protein, and vitamins. And people say vegans are deprived?

$1^3/_4$ cups organic apple juice or Rejuvelac (page XX)

1 frozen banana (peel before freezing)

2 tablespoons lecithin granules

2 tablespoons Karyn's Kare Green Meal Powder

2 tablespoons flaxseed oil or coconut oil

Combine the juice and banana in a blender and process until smooth. Add the lecithin and process briefly. Add the Green Meal Powder and oil and process on low to medium speed until well combined. Pour and enjoy!

TIPS

- High-quality organic apple juice should appear cloudy. Clear apple juice has been filtered to extend its shelf life, and this process greatly reduces the amount of healthful polyphenols and antioxidants in the juice.
- Use more apple juice for a sweeter shake.
- During your cleanse, follow the recipe as written. However, when you're not detoxing, feel free to adapt it to make it your own. Use almond milk or hemp milk instead of apple juice, blueberries or pineapple instead of banana, and hemp oil instead of flaxseed oil. There are so many ways to shake up this shake. Keep it interesting!

Smooth Move with Spirulina

This delicious and creamy smoothie is chock-full of vitamins, minerals, and essential fatty acids. It also is a great way to use up any leftover flaxseeds or spirulina you may have after the cleanse.

1 cup nut milk

1 frozen banana (peel before freezing)

1/2 cup coconut water

2 tablespoons cold-milled organic flaxseed powder

1 teaspoon spirulina powder

1/2 teaspoon vanilla extract

Put the nut milk, banana, coconut water, flaxseed powder, and vanilla extract in a blender and process on low speed until combined. Add the spirulina powder and pulse a few times until fully incorporated. Serve immediately.

Flaxseed Cereal

Flaxseeds are an excellent source of omega-3 fatty acids and fiber, and this simple cereal is a terrific way to get them into your diet.

2 tablespoons cold-milled organic flaxseed powder

6 tablespoons coconut water

½ banana, chopped

½ teaspoon ground cinnamon

Combine the flaxseed powder and coconut water in a bowl. Let sit for about 10 minutes, until the flaxseed powder has absorbed some of the liquid and softened. Add the banana and cinnamon and stir to combine. Serve immediately.

TIP: This recipe is endlessly adaptable. Experiment by adding your favorite fruits, green powders, or spices.

Raw Oatmeal

Here is a raw twist on a familiar, quick, and satisfying breakfast food. Vary it by adding different spices and fruits.

1 cup oat groats

2½ cups organic apple juice

1 apple, chopped

¼ cup raisins

¼ cup agave nectar or other sweetener

Soak the groats in the juice for about 3 hours, or until the juice is mostly absorbed. Stir in the apple, raisins, and agave nectar. Serve immediately.

TIPS

- Add ground cinnamon or other sweet spices to taste.
- Vary the recipe by using other fresh and dried fruits.

Dr. Wigmore's Energy Soup

Energy Soup is a complete meal that provides most of the vitamins and nutrients you need for the day.

1 1/2 cups Rejuvelac (page 106)

1 teaspoon dulse flakes

1 to 2 apples, coarsely chopped

1 cup baby spinach leaves

1/4 to 1/2 cup sunflower sprouts

1/4 to 1/2 cup buckwheat sprouts (optional)

1 avocado

Combine the Rejuvelac and dulse in a blender and process for about 30 seconds. Add the apples and pulse to combine. Add the spinach and pulse until chopped. Add the sunflower sprouts and optional buckwheat sprouts and pulse until coarsely chopped. Add the avocado and pulse until the soup is the desired consistency. Pour into a beautiful bowl and serve. Stored in a sealed glass container in the refrigerator, Dr. Wigmore's Energy Soup will keep for 7 to 10 days.

TIPS

- Use a high-powered blender, such as a Vitamix, with a variable-speed dial.
- For some people, Dr. Wigmore's Energy Soup is an acquired taste. Tweak the ingredients and amounts to your taste.
- If you like savory seasonings, add cayenne, garlic, and sea salt to taste.
- If you don't have sunflower and buckwheat sprouts on hand, use any other sprouted greens you have.
- Make a double batch of soup and store it in the refrigerator to use throughout the week. The soup will expand, so store it in a glass container, not plastic.

Almond Pâté

Pâté is a versatile staple of the raw diet. Change the veggies and seasonings to vary the taste and create different ethnic recipes.

2 cups almonds

4 cups purified water

1 beefsteak or other tomato

$1/4$ small white onion

3 to 4 tablespoons Bragg Liquid Aminos

2 cloves garlic

$1/4$ teaspoon cayenne

Soak the almonds in the water for 8 to 12 hours.

Drain and rinse the almonds. Transfer the almonds to a food processor and pulse a few times, just until coarsely chopped. Add the tomato, onion, Bragg Liquid Aminos, garlic, and cayenne. Process until the desired consistency is achieved. Stored in a glass container in the refrigerator, Almond Pâté will keep for 7 to 10 days.

TIPS

- For a creamier pâté, add a small amount of avocado.
- If you don't finish the pâté in 7 to 10 days, spread it on dehydrator trays and dehydrate it into crackers. The crackers will keep indefinitely.

MOCK TUNA SALAD: Add dulse flakes and chopped celery to taste.

Cashew Sour Cream

A fermented living food that is full of beneficial bacteria, this raw sour cream can be used in parfaits, sandwiches, smoothies, and soups. The possibilities are endless.

4 cups cashews

1 1/2 cups Rejuvelac (page 106)

Put the cashews in a medium bowl and cover with purified water. Let rest in a cool place or in the refrigerator for 8 to 12 hours.

Drain the cashews in a colander and rinse them until the water runs clear. Transfer to a blender and add the Rejuvelac. Process until smooth and creamy; the mixture will be thick. Pour into a clean glass jar and cover the top with cheesecloth (use a string or rubber band to keep it secure).

Let stand in a warm place (72 to 78 degrees F) for 48 hours. When bubbles or air pockets start to form, scoop off and discard the top layer of the mixture (it will be brown due to oxidation). Transfer to a clean glass jar and seal. Stored in the refrigerator, Cashew Sour Cream will keep for 4 weeks.

Karyn's Lemon-Herb Dressing

No one would ever guess that this creamy, delicious dressing is vegan and raw. Use it on salads or serve it as a party dip to impress your friends.

1 cup extra-virgin olive oil

$1/2$ cup freshly squeezed lemon juice

$1/2$ cups cider vinegar

1 cup purified water

$1/2$ cup Bragg Liquid Aminos

$1/3$ cup agave nectar or other sweetener

$1/4$ cup peeled garlic cloves

1 teaspoon sea salt

$3/4$ teaspoon dried basil

$3/4$ teaspoon dried dill weed

$3/4$ tablespoon dried oregano

$3/4$ teaspoon dried rosemary

$3/4$ teaspoon dried thyme

Pinch dried bay leaf

1 tablespoon dulse flakes

Combine the oil and lemon juice in a blender and process on the lowest speed. With the blender running, adding the ingredients in this order through the cap opening in the lid: vinegar, water, Bragg Liquid Aminos, agave nectar, garlic, salt, basil, dill weed, oregano, rosemary, thyme, and bay leaf. Turn off the blender. Add the dulse and pulse just until it is evenly distributed. Stored in a sealed glass jar in the refrigerator, Karyn's Lemon-Herb Dressing will keep for 4 weeks.

Berry-Flax Parfait

This parfait is an easy-to-make and healthful dessert. It's also a great snack when you're craving something sweet.

2 cups raw cashews

$1/4$ cup agave nectar or other sweetener

1 cup cold-milled organic flaxseed powder

$1^1/_2$ cups thinly sliced strawberries

To make a cashew cream, put the cashews in a medium bowl and cover with purified water. Let soak for 6 to 8 hours.

Drain the cashews in a colander and rinse. Transfer to a blender. Add the agave nectar and begin processing. With the blender running, add just enough purified water through the cap opening in the lid to create a creamy consistency. Process until smooth.

For each parfait, put a dollop of the cashew cream in a decorative glass. Top with 1 tablespoon of the flaxseed powder and a thin layer of the strawberries. Make another layer using ¼ cup of the cashew cream, 1 tablespoon of the flaxseed powder, and another layer of the strawberries. Repeat once more, finishing with a layer of the strawberries and a sprinkle of the flaxseed powder. Serve immediately, or cover and refrigerate for up to 48 hours.

This cleanse has opened my eyes to the world we live in. Convenience stores are filled with alcohol, candy, cigarettes, soda, snacks, and other crap. Fast food restaurants are everywhere. Where is the good nutritional stuff? I have become a more disciplined person, eating right, in this insane world. It feels amazing! This cleanse also eliminated some emotional weight I've been carrying. I'm not sure how or why, but this detox has definitely helped my self-confidence level. The world needs more Karyns.

—J. L.

Since taking the class, I have found it much easier to eat raw food all day, every day. My skin looks better, my stomach is flatter, my body is leaner, and I am sleeping better. I'm way more relaxed, even at work. I feel strong, athletic, and self-confident. —J.

Since completing the program, I feel more grounded, more centered, and more complete. I will always remember what Karyn says about the program: "It's just 28 short days, and it's no more trouble than doing chemotherapy." —M.

You cannot help but be inspired by Karyn's beauty: her clear, sparkling eyes; cocoa-colored, flawless skin; youthful energy; and slim, statuesque figure. She reminds us of what is available to all—if we choose to nurture our bodies with raw food, proper exercise, and prayer. It is comforting to know that there is a place to go where everyone is welcomed with open arms, no judgment, and coaching from the heart by a human being who holds her clients as friends and always sees them in their highest potential light. —S. B.

I am still eating raw food, and I feel wonderful. I am also still losing weight. I never thought I would say this, but I hope it stops soon! My blood pressure is in the normal range and my cholesterol has dropped. The doctor told me to just keep doing what I'm doing. I can't tell you how happy I am that I decided to do the detoxification program! —E. C.

When I began my journey with the detox class, my primary goals were to reclaim and revitalize my health by eliminating excess weight and lowering my high blood pressure and high cholesterol. I strongly believe that I am already healed. I am very grateful to have made a lifetime commitment to honoring the gift of life and healthy choices.

—D. R.

I had just quit drinking four months prior to the class, so it couldn't have come along at a better time. I've learned a lot about how I want to eat and how I want my body to work. I feel much more aware, both physically and spiritually. I would recommend this class to all I know and love.

—M. A. C.

The class is an excellent starting point for anyone who wishes to improve his or her overall health. The instructions are easy to follow and logical.

—D. M.

We spend a lot of time cleaning the outside of our bodies but forget about cleaning the inside. Even though I have been a vegetarian for many years, this cleanse was a good rest for my body from many bad foods besides meat. I would recommend it for everyone.

—K. C.

The emotional impact of the detox was just as intense if not more intense than the physical impact. It was as though many of the emotions and thoughts that I had been trying to suppress needed to come out— and they did. I view this cleanse as a stepping stone to a lifetime of health and vitality.

—A. S.

resources

ORDERING PRODUCTS AND STAYING IN TOUCH

Karyn's Fresh Corner
1901 N. Halsted Street
Chicago, IL 60614
312-255-1590

www.karynraw.com
karyninfo@karynraw.com
twitter @KarynCalabrese
*Follow us on Facebook
and twitter @KarynsRawBeauty*

NETWORK WITH OTHER DETOXERS AND SHARE COMMENTS AND QUESTIONS:

www.karynraw.com/detoxcommunity

KARYN'S OTHER RESTAURANTS

Karyn's Cooked
738 N. Wells Street
Chicago, IL 60654
312-587-1050
www.karynraw.com

Karyn's on Green
130 S. Green Street
Chicago, IL 60607
312-226-6155
www.karynsongreen.com
*Follow us on Facebook
and twitter @karynsongreen*

SPROUTMAN WHEATGRASS

Fresh wheatgrass or freshly frozen wheatgrass juice, shipped overnight to
the United States or Canada.

P.O. Box 1100
Great Barrington, MA 01230

413-528-5200, ext. 2
www.sproutman.com

RAW VEGAN RECIPE BOOKS

Hooked on Raw by Rhio
Living Raw Food by Sarma Melngailis
Raw by Charlie Trotter and Roxanne Klein
Raw Food Made Easy for 1 or 2 People by Jennifer Cornbleet

Raw Food/Real World by Matthew Kenney and Sarma Melngailis
Raw for Dessert by Jennifer Cornbleet
Raw: The UNcook Book by Juliano Brotman and Erika Lenkert
The Raw 50 by Carol Alt
The Raw Food Revolution Diet by Cherie Soria, Brenda Davis, RD, and Vesanto Melina, MS, RD

COOKED VEGAN RECIPE BOOKS

Great Chefs Cook Vegan by Linda Long
Vegan Lunch Box by Jennifer McCann
Vegan Soul Kitchen by Bryant Terry
Vegan with a Vengeance and other books by Isa Chandra Moskowitz
Veganomicon by Isa Chandra Moskowitz and Terry Hope Romero

OTHER GREAT BOOKS ABOUT RAW FOOD AND HEALTH

Any books by Gabriel Cousens, MD
Breaking the Death Habit by Leonard Orr
Coconut Oil for Health and Beauty by Cynthia and Laura Holzapfel
Fasting by Allan Cott, MD
Sprouts the Miracle Food by Steve Meyerowitz
Survival in the 21st Century by Viktoras Kulvinskas
The Cancer Cure that Worked by Barry Lynes
The China Study by T. Colin Campbell
The Coconut Oil Miracle by Bruce Fife, CN, ND
The Sprouting Book and any other books by Ann Wigmore
Thrive and *Thrive Fitness* by Brendan Brazier

INSPIRATIONAL READS (GREAT WHILE FASTING)

365 Science of Mind by Ernest Holmes
God Spoke to Me by Eileen Caddy
The Essene Gospel of Peace by Edmond Bordeaux Szekely
The Golden Present by Swami Satchidananda

INFORMATION ABOUT THE ANIMAL AGRICULTURE INDUSTRY

Eating Animals by Jonathan Safran Foer
Food, Inc. (book and movie)
Peaceable Kingdom (movie)
The Future of Food (movie)
World Peace Diet by Will M. Tuttle, PhD

The program has been perhaps as intellectually enlightening as it has been physically enlightening. I am learning to rethink everything I've been taught about food over the course of my lifetime. I'm understanding that most food meets more of a social need than a physiological one. I'm also seeing how well the body responds to being treated right. It's quite an awakening! I will never again think of food the same way. I'm ready to approach the "buffet of life" with a much more selective and educated palate and the ability to make wiser choices about what to put on my plate.

—K. V.

I occasionally worry about getting diabetes, like my mother, but I know that if I stay with this new lifestyle, I will lessen the possibility of that occurring.

—C. L.

Wow! Where do I begin? I feel light. I feel clear. I feel balanced. I am in touch with my body. The detoxification class gave me the understanding and awareness that what I choose to eat and drink at any moment has a profound effect on how I will feel. In addition, everyone is telling me how great I look!

—T. W.

Here I am, craving wheatgrass juice, vegetable juice, and rejuvelac, not just because they're good for me, but for the way they make me feel. If I had known this change in my diet would make me feel this good, I would have done it years ago. My thoughts are much clearer, my creativity at work has increased, and I feel fantastic! It has only been three weeks, and I can't wait to see how good I will feel in another three weeks.

—M. A. B.

Taking this class has been the next step in my quest for better health and disease prevention.
                                                                        —J. M. C.

Since this was my first cleanse, I had no expectation in terms of results. I've achieved clarity, balance, the satisfaction of knowing I can accomplish whatever goals I set for myself, and a true sense of self-reliance. Additionally, I'm much more aware and concerned about what I'm putting into my body (as well as what I'm putting on it). This class is a great catalyst for anyone interested in improving his or her health and life.
                                                                        —J. T.

The detox program gave me a physical, spiritual, emotional, and mental awakening. I will forever be thankful and blessed because of it.
                                                                        —B. B.

This is the first detox I have ever been on, and I can see what a difference it has created in my body. I have hypoglycemia, and I used to eat every time I started feeling shaky and weak. Since the detox program, my blood sugar has become very stable.
                                                                        —L. B.

I was tempted to quit after the first week, but I am glad I continued because the results are fantastic!
                                                                        —T. D.

index

References for sidebars, testimony, and the names of recipes appear in *italic* typeface.

cracker/bread recommendations, 39

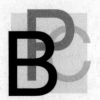

BOOK PUBLISHING COMPANY

since 1974—books that educate, inspire, and empower

To find sprouting seeds and other vegan favorites online, visit:
www.healthy-eating.com

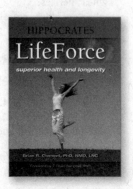

Hippocrates LifeForce

Brian R. Clement, PhD, NMD, LNC

978-1-57067-249-1 $14.95

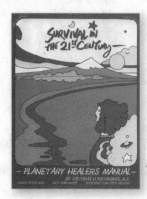

Survival in the 21st Century

Viktoras H. Kulvinskas

978-1-57067-247-7 $29.95

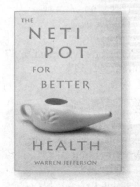

The Neti Pot for Better Health

Warren Jefferson

978-1-57067-186-9 $9.95

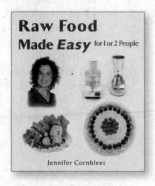

Raw Food Made Easy

Jennifer Cornbleet

978-1-57067-175-3 $17.95

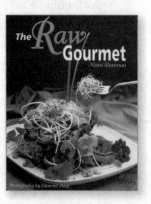

The Raw Gourmet

Nomi Shannon

978-0-92047-048-0 $24.95

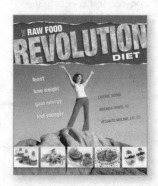

The Raw Food Revolution Diet

Cherie Soria,
Brenda Davis, RD,
Vesanto Melina, MS, RD

978-1-57067-185-2 $21.95

Purchase these health titles and cookbooks from your local bookstore or natural food store,
or you can buy them directly from:

Book Publishing Company • P.O. Box 99 • Summertown, TN 38483 • 1-800-695-2241

Please include $3.95 per book for shipping and handling.

"After taking Karyn's detox class and following her program, I am more energetic and have better digestion and improved immune function (no colds or flu). During the detox program, I witnessed and was impressed by how many individuals in her class experienced rapid changes in their health. For example, people with high blood pressure were able to lower it, diabetics reduced their need for insulin, and those with digestive problems improved significantly. Karyn's program has changed many people's lives by educating and motivating them to take control of their health."

Dorothy Anasinski, DDS

"As a medical doctor, I am impressed by Karyn's knowledge, because it is medically sound as well as practical and useful. I followed her program almost 100 percent with unbelievable results, including having energy for eighteen-hour days full of patient, family, and personal responsibilities; no more annoying cravings for sugar; the disappearance of lifelong skin issues; improved clarity of thinking; and increased happiness and confidence.

I also learned about a world of health products I was not aware of. I am particularly impressed by Karyn's private-label products. I have confidence in their efficacy and have had great results using them. In fact, I carry her products in my office and often prescribe them to patients. I strongly recommend the use of the Green Kamut Powder, Green Meal Powder, Systemic Enzymes, and Digestive Enzymes. I also encourage my patients to take a detox class."

Lorene Wu, MD, Dipl. Ac.

"Karyn has succeeded in writing one of the most comprehensive vegan nutrition books, which acknowledges the relationship between a healthy body temple and one's inner spirit. Raising a fork of Karyn's food is an invitation to a sacred feast that awakens and nourishes the spiritual senses. I thank the Natural World for the sustenance it gives us through her culinary creations."

Michael Bernard Beckwith
author, *Spiritual Liberation: Fulfilling Your Soul's Potential*

The first time I walked into Karyn's restaurant in Chicago, it was love at first sight. And the food is delicious too! I felt safe, healthy, and fulfilled. This is all due to Karyn's vision.

John Salley
owner, John Salley Foods; former NBA star

"Karyn has no doubt crafted a bestseller with *Soak Your Nuts*. Her personalized journey into healing has brought even more meaning to her delicious recipes and vibrant theory. I was captivated while reading her story, from her trials of illness and imbalance to her recovery. I was spellbound by her awareness of our current environmental and health crisis as well as her ability to remain positive and hopeful for a better future. She is a vigilant steward of the planet and an inspirational healer. Hers is truly an evolutionary work of creativity, wisdom, and intelligence."

Juliano
author, *Raw: The UNcook Book*